44½ Cl you can make if you have cancer

How To Take Control Of Your Illness

SHEILA DAINOW

VICKI GOLDING

JO WRIGHT

Newleaf

Newleaf
an imprint of
Gill & Macmillan Ltd
Hume Avenue
Park West
Dublin 12
with associated companies throughout the world
www.gillmacmillan.ie

Print origination by O'K Graphic Design, Dublin

Printed by
ColourBooks Ltd, Dublin

1 3 5 4 2

This book is dedicated to

Barry who died unexpectedly before the book was published. His love meant so much to me then and will always remain with me. (Vicki)

Simon who laughed and cried with me and is my soul mate. (Jo)

Cyril generous as always with love and care. (Sheila)

Contents

Introduction

ↄ⊁⊰∾

Acknowledgments

This is our opportunity to thank those people who have supported us through our experience of cancer and helped in the writing of this book

Firstly, a very special mention to Lesley Fuentes who was so generous in sharing her own experience and contributed greatly to the finished manuscript.

We also appreciate those who contributed their voices to the book: Cyril Dainow, Alisa Dolev, Jillian Dunstan, Laura Golding, Anne Imbabi, Simon Nicholson and Barry Roddy.

Special thanks to Nan, Noreen, Michael, Rosemary and Jane who were unstinting with loving support.

We were also greatly supported by our work colleagues at Edmonton and Southgate Home Care Team and other colleagues at Enfield Social Services.

We value highly the expertise, care and ongoing support shown by our medical practitioners, particularly Dr Elaine Yeo, Mr Qureshi, Dr Sivananthan and Professor Ian Jacobs.

Thanks are also due to our agent Carole Blake for her

tireless support and guidance and to Michael Gill for his constructive and helpful advice.

Last, but definitely not least, are the many friends and family who helped us through our illness. To have experienced that quality of love and care has been a wonderful privilege.

Foreword

Most of us have a deep fear of developing cancer but a limited understanding of what it really means or how we would cope with it. Unfortunately, the diagnosis of cancer arrives for more than a third of us at some point during our lifetime. Even if we are fortunate enough to avoid cancer ourselves, most of us will at some point be deeply affected by cancer in a friend, colleague or close relative. When the diagnosis arrives, it is inevitably a time of turmoil that very few of us are well prepared for. How can we cope and who should we turn to for support and to answer our questions? Even the best doctors and nurses are only with their patients for a small portion of the time and are inevitably focusing their efforts on the details of medical care and treatment. Relatives and friends may care desperately but will usually have little experience and may also have difficulty coping. This book provides a wonderful combination of practical and emotional advice for patients and those close to them about how to cope with a diagnosis of cancer and its aftermath.

The book is written by Jo and Vicki, who have been through the turmoil of a cancer diagnosis and their mother/friend, Sheila, who has supported them and also has broad experience of counselling. The combination of personal and professional experience has enabled them to produce a unique book, which tackles the difficult issues raised by a diagnosis of cancer. The result is an invaluable guide not only for patients themselves but also for those closest to them. The style of the book makes it accessible as a reference, to dip into for specific questions, or to read from start to finish as an overall guide to the cancer journey. There are sections on questions every cancer patient has to tackle: Who to tell? What to read? What questions to ask your doctor? How should you expect to feel? Is it okay to get another opinion? Is it all right to cry and to laugh? How can you cope with worry, fear and panic? Is it okay to feel down? What should you expect from other people's responses? The book also provides guidance on numerous practical issues including: finding support from patient groups and counsellors; strategies for staying in control; what to expect from the hospital and treatment; how to cope with change in appearance; returning home and returning to work; making sense of your life and other priorities; how to handle your friends, family and partner; and taking care of yourself.

A great deal of vital work is currently underway to improve the care of patients with cancer. This involves prevention, screening, reducing delays in diagnosis, ensuring a uniformly high standard of treatment and making sure that supportive care is widely available. Even when all of these important advances have been made, patients with cancer will still face the difficult issues addressed in this book. I am sure that most doctors and nurses involved in cancer care share my frustration with the limits to which we are able to help patients with these questions and problems. A brief appointment every few weeks doesn't leave much time to discuss the questions in this book, particularly when most of the time is needed for examination and treatment planning. Even patients looked after in the most caring and well organised cancer centres have to tackle many of the issues raised in this book relying largely on their own resources and the support of those closest to them. This book will help them to cope with their cancer and will reassure them that the feelings and problems it poses are 'normal'. It will be a great help to have it available for patients.

I was part of the team who looked after Jo and helped her to deal with the difficult decisions and emotions, which along with the experience of Vicki and Sheila inspired this book. It was a privilege to take care of Jo and it is an honour to have contributed in a small way to the production of this book. I know that it will help many patients and those closest to them to cope with the trauma of a cancer diagnosis.

Ian Jacobs,
Professor of Gynaecological Oncology,
St Bartholomew's Hospital, London
President, British Gynaecological Cancer Society

Introduction

This is a book that is meant to be *used*; to be kept by your side rather than on the bookshelf. It is a guide to the emotional and practical problems which arise for cancer sufferers and for their nearest and dearest. In it you will find suggestions which are designed to help you through some of the difficulties you might be facing; to give you choices where you thought there might be none.

Our aim is to help you make the most of your life, whatever your situation; to see some light where you thought there was only darkness; even to smile when you thought you never would again.

The book is not a definitive text about cancer and its treatment; it cannot be a substitute for medical or psychological therapy. However, it can be a constant companion ready to be 'dipped into' whenever the going gets tough.

We know that this is not what you planned for the next part of your life. It might seem like a time when all your choice has been taken away. However, from our experience we know that there are choices you can make at each stage that may help you through.

The book is in four sections:

- Pre-diagnosis

- Diagnosis

- Treatment

- The aftermath

Each section describes the choices available to you and offers suggestions as to how you might make the most of your situation.

You will meet the authors of the book through excerpts from their diaries and memories. They are Vicki Golding, Jo Wright and Sheila Dainow.

Vicki Golding (61) was a manager for social services for 13 years and is now a social-work consultant. She had a mastectomy in 1992 following a diagnosis of breast cancer. She set up the first workplace cancer support group in England and is currently a member of CancerLife, a cancer service users' project.

Jo Wright (34) currently works as a home care manager for a local authority. She has recently become a voluntary area Fone Friend co-ordinator for Ovacome (the ovarian cancer network charity). She was diagnosed with ovarian cancer in

Introduction

༺❀༻

November 1997. She had four operations in less than a year and now her doctor is optimistic that the cancer has physically gone although she is still working through the psychological aftermath.

Sheila Dainow (61) (Jo's mother/Vicki's friend) has worked as a counsellor and trainer with groups and individuals for over thirty years. She is a member of the Society of Holistic Practitioners and a Fellow of the British Association for Counselling. She has been writing since 1985 and brings to this book the particular experience of the 'onlooker' trying to support loved ones through the problems of serious illness.

You will also 'meet' some of the people who were most closely involved and who share their thoughts and feelings as their memories of that time appear throughout the book.

They are:

Cyril Dainow: Jo's dad

Alisa Dolev: Jo's sister who lives abroad

Jillian Dunstan: Vicki's elder daughter

Laura Golding: Vicki's younger daughter/ Jo's friend

Anne Imbabi: Jo's friend and manager

Simon Nicholson: Jo's partner

Barry Roddy: Vicki's partner

Having any serious illness is like embarking on a journey into unknown territory. At times it will seem dangerous and difficult. A good map is one that could ease a journey into the unknown. Of course, we don't have the map of *your* particular journey but we do have our own and we hope that at times you will find it of help in pointing out the way.

Section 1 Pre-diagnosis

'Have I? Haven't I?'

Choice 1

Move Out Of Limbo

Doubt is the beginning, not the end, of wisdom.

Sir Walter Scott (1771–1832)

You are worried because you have found a lump, unexpected bleeding or another symptom which makes you think you might have cancer. What can you do?

One choice you have is, of course, to ignore your symptoms. At first it can seem more comfortable to stay in limbo; not knowing means you can pretend all is well.

But …

- As long as you stay in limbo your imagination is free to run riot and your fears increase.

- If you do have cancer it might be harder to cure if it is treated later rather than earlier.

- Ignoring something does not make it go away.

So …

- Make the move out of limbo, into action. Visit your general practitioner or health centre to discuss your symptoms. This may seem like a risky thing to do because you are facing up to the fact that you might have cancer. On the other hand there might be another explanation for your symptoms and you may be worrying unnecessarily.

- If you want some information or advice before you do this, you can contact one of the many organisations that are there to help you (see list at end of book).

I found the lump in October. I went to my GP expecting to be reassured that it was nothing serious as had happened on other occasions. Ten days later I saw the senior registrar who told me there was a 50 per cent chance I had cancer. Not knowing whether I had cancer meant that my life was at a standstill. I could think of nothing else. I longed to escape from myself but there was no way out. —Vicki

Choice 2

Being Afraid Does Not Mean You Are Helpless

Fear of danger is ten thousand times more terrifying than danger itself.

Daniel Defoe (1661–1731)

If your general practitioner is concerned about your symptoms you are likely to be referred to a consultant. You can also expect to have a series of tests and/or scans. While you wait for these appointments you can feel as if you're on a seesaw – when you're 'up' you can be optimistic; when you're 'down' you can be full of fears. Time can hang heavily on your hands.

Living with fear is like having a dark cloud over your mind. Sometimes this cloud is all-enveloping, at other times just a shadow on the sun. If you do have times when you feel overwhelmed, maybe these suggestions will help you to stop fear being in control all the time.

❧ Think of how you have handled fears in the past and overcome them. Use those methods now.

∾ Feel OK about whatever you are feeling. It's absolutely normal to feel angry, scared, worried, disbelieving, numb or shocked in this situation. You don't have to add to your fear by wondering if you are going mad.

∾ You can also feel OK about your positive feelings. There will be times when you forget your worries and have a good laugh; in fact the more you can do this, the better for your mind and body.

∾ Don't ignore what your body tells you. Worry can be very draining, so if you feel exhausted in the middle of the day take a rest.

∾ Try the Ten-Minute Worry Plan. It is difficult to stop worrying when we are afraid of what the future may hold. The problem with this is that worrying does not actually change anything other than making us feel worse. You can prove this to yourself. Choose a convenient ten-minute slot when you can be on your own and worry. Don't think about anything else except how worried you are. When the ten minute slot is up, check to see whether anything has actually changed. Of course, apart from having used up ten minutes of time, everything is just the same. So if you are a natural worrier it is worth trying to find a way to control these thoughts. You could try allocating a particular time each day as 'worry time'. If you find yourself feeling frightened at other times, try telling yourself that you can think about that at the chosen time and get on with something else.

- Try to arrange things so that you are not often on your own. Being with people you like will help you to feel more safe and secure.

- Write down your thoughts because sometimes things seem less frightening once they are written down.

- Carry out whatever plans you have made – theatre visits, dinner parties, holidays and so on. You may not enjoy them as much as you would if you weren't anxious, but they will give you some relief from being alone with your thoughts.

- If you have a confidante, talk about your fears; cry if you feel like it.

- You can distract yourself by watching TV; it can be harder to concentrate on a book.

- Treat yourself kindly; this is a time when you are vulnerable and need looking after. Rest; have long, scented baths letting the water wash over you; allow time to slip away. Using a relaxation tape may help you to be more at peace with yourself.

- ❧ Your general practitioner can be a good source of support and may well be able to tell you about hypnotherapy, self-hypnosis, visualisation, meditation and so on.

The whole world is a very narrow bridge, and the important thing is not to be afraid.

Attributed to Nachman of Bratzlav (1772–1811)

It was during this time that I started to realise how lucky I was. I know that sounds strange but the impact of realising that had we not gone for fertility treatment nothing would have been discovered until it was probably too late to treat, was massive.

—Jo

Choice 3

To Tell Or Not To Tell

A trouble shared is a trouble halved.

Proverb

Facing fear on your own can be a very lonely experience. One of the choices you have at this time is whether to confide in someone or keep your fears to yourself until you are certain about the situation. The decision to tell your close family and friends has pros and cons.

Pros

- Everyone knows where they stand. You don't have to hide your emotions and pretend everything is OK when it isn't.

- It will be easier for you to ask for help.

- Other people tend to keep you more in touch with reality, curbing the worst fears that may be rampaging around in your mind.

- It may help you to prepare others for what may be to come.

- Those close to you will feel trusted.

- If you don't tell people they may say, 'Why didn't you tell me?' because all they want to do is offer love and support.

Cons

- You may find yourself having to cope with the fears of the people in whom you confide. They may find it difficult to hear what you are saying and try to discount your fears, or they may want more information than you are prepared to give.

- People may not know what to say or they may have too much to say (especially about the grim side).

- You may feel you are burdening the people who are close to you by telling them of your fears.

- If you want your environment to remain as routine as possible it may be more difficult for you to feel ordinary and be treated 'normally' if all those around you know what you are worried about.

❦

> *I felt anxious waiting for the results of Mum's biopsy. I tried not to think about the possibility that she might have breast cancer and tried instead to focus on the often-quoted statistic that most breast lumps are benign. I felt increasingly worried as the day of the results drew closer and had a sense of foreboding. I remember feeling pleased that I was working that day so I could be distracted from my worries. I remember all day waiting for that phone call.* — Laura

If you do decide to tell, it is important to confide in people you trust; people who will listen to what you are feeling and who will be able to offer support.

If you don't want to confide in anyone you know at this point you might want to ring a helpline run by one of the cancer organisations (see list at end of book), arrange to see a counsellor or talk to a minister of religion.

You may be wondering whether to inform your place of work. Once again there are pros and cons.

Pros

❧ You won't need to hide your vulnerability all the time and find explanations for times when you find it hard to concentrate or feel weepy.

✒ You can be open about needing time for hospital appointments.

> *I know that Jo is strong but was she put under stress at work over the years? Did I add to her stress when I was teaching her the business?* —Anne

Cons

✒ You may feel your job would be threatened.

✒ It may not be appropriate to discuss personal aspects of your life with colleagues.

In general, our experience is that sharing your fears is beneficial. It takes a lot of mental energy to keep fear under control, so communicating your feelings tends to leave you feeling relieved of some of the pressure afterwards. Although you don't want the whole world to know, confiding in one or two people who care about you or who have been through the same experience can be very therapeutic.

Choice 4

To Read Or Not To Read

While you are waiting for your various appointments you might feel like looking up everything you can about the type of cancer you think you might have. Reading can be helpful; in any bookshop or library you will find a range of literature on the subject. Most of the organisations quoted at the end of the book publish information leaflets.

But … some words of warning!

❧ The trouble with reading articles and medical books about cancer is that they can be very frightening. People do die of cancer and you may be worried that you have a particular cancer which has a poor survival rate. Remember, though, that you have not yet been diagnosed with cancer and you could be worrying needlessly.

❧ Beware of statistics! Until you actually have your diagnosis you will not know what information is relevant to you. The implications of statistics are best explained by a consultant who can help you relate them to your particular situation. For example, in most cases, if cancer is caught at an early stage, prognosis is better than if it is detected late.

Cancer seemed all around me. Newspaper headlines screamed out about the latest famous person to die of cancer, about new shock statistics linking everyday food to cancer, 10 symptoms that mean you have cancer ... the word cancer always seemed to occur in the same sentence as 'terminally ill', 'dying' and 'died'. Somehow that week I did not notice the hopeful stories about survivors of cancer, new cures and so on. — Laura

---

- Some cancer sufferers have written inspiring accounts of their experience and it can be helpful to know how others coped. However, these tales can be depressing and feed your fears at this stage, especially if the person has not survived. While these books are sometimes cathartic for the author they may not support the reader. Choose carefully.

- You will notice that since you became worried, every soap opera, film, radio programme, magazine article and newspaper will carry a story on just the kind of cancer you are worried about (and often with a bad diagnosis to step up the drama). It's a bit like learning a new word and then finding it all over the place even though you never noticed it before. It may feel like these programmes and articles are aimed at you personally but they really aren't; you are just more sensitive to the subject.

I didn't set out to read anything special but I read the newspaper. Just like when you split up from a partner you only hear sad songs, there seemed to be an article on cancer in the paper every day. — Simon

Obviously it is up to you to choose what to read at this stage; we would recommend caution until you know what your condition is. It is very difficult to read a book that describes symptoms, without immediately feeling every single one of them! You won't be able to accurately diagnose your own illness at this stage.

I frightened myself by reading articles about breast cancer, which quoted figures of 25,000 cases and 11,000 deaths a year. Each time I came across an article, I froze. Everything I read depressed me. — Vicki

A witty statesman said, you might prove anything by figures.
Thomas Carlyle (1795–1881)

Choice 5

❦

Testing Times

Patience is a virtue.
Proverb

If your doctor or consultant thinks that you might have cancer you are likely to have a series of tests and/or scans which may include a blood test, x-rays, bone scan, liver ultrasound and so on. These tests can be scary. You may feel very lonely and vulnerable having your body scanned, however kind the medical staff are. Each test brings you nearer to facing the possibility of illness so naturally you will feel nervous.

❧ Don't be afraid to ask for specific details of the actual tests you are having. Find out why the tests are being done, what will actually happen and when you will know the results. Occasionally you might be told a result immediately, but it is more usual to have to wait for the results.

❧ Many of the tests are not physically painful at all, but they can be emotionally draining. So it's a good idea to take someone with you to be there for you during and after the procedures. If you can, programme some rest time for yourself after the test.

- Be prepared for long waits and try not to get too wound-up while you are waiting. Take some things to help you pass the time such as a good book or magazine, a Walkman, knitting or crochet.

- If you don't feel too confident about asking questions, brief your companion to ask for you.

> *I was pleased to be able to go with Jo to some of her appointments. We were able to talk afterwards about it and check what we'd understood. It also made me feel that I could do something positive, better than just sitting at home waiting and worrying.* — Sheila

- Be sure to check whether any preparation is necessary; do you have to fast for a number of hours before the test, for example?

- Tests can be scary. Creating the image of a place or the sound of music or a song you particularly like and keeping that in your mind can help you through.

> *The test I found most scary was the MRI scan. It wasn't painful but I felt unprepared for the claustrophobic feeling and the noise. No one had explained to me what to expect.*
>
> —Jo

It is natural to be anxious about the results of the tests, but each one means you are moving forward — away from the unknown.

Choice 6

❦

Don't Stop

'Tain't no use to sit and whine
'Cause the fish ain't on your line
Bait your hook an' keep on tryin', keep agoin'.

Frank L. Stanton (1857–1927)

It is important to continue your normal life while everything is so uncertain. You may find it hard to think about anything except cancer but you will feel better if you manage to keep going.

- ❧ Go to work but accept that it may be difficult to concentrate.

- ❧ Eat good food. This is a time when you may need comfort so why not 'comfort eat' if it helps you feel better? Have a drink – but not too much alcohol as its ultimate effect is to depress.

- ❧ Continue to carry out any practical plans you had made.

> *We were in the middle of decorating our home. It gave me a real boost looking at what we had done and I wanted to complete it.* —Vicki

- Buy something new – clothes, a hat, scented body care – anything that will give you a lift.

- Sleep when you need to.

- You may find that you have become self-absorbed; little things may irritate you. This is natural.

- At those times when you feel you just can't cope, it is not a weakness to allow other people to take over if they are around. It is a strength to be able to know when 'enough's enough' and be able to say so. Let someone else decide what to have for dinner, cook and wash up, decide which film to see and so on.

- Rest when you need to. Don't feel guilty about doing nothing. You need to recover from the emotional trauma and build up your strength for what is to come.

- You may find you keep going over things. What if … ? What did I do wrong? Was it an accident? What if I had eaten different food? And so on. This constant going over and over things you might have done differently doesn't change or improve anything. Find some mental relaxation that allows you to silence the chatterbox in your head.

> *I wanted to watch programmes with happy endings and no mention of illness so I borrowed some Walt Disney videos from my niece. Watching them allowed me to escape for a couple of hours.* —Jo

You may be surprised to find that even though you are scared about the future you can still enjoy things and even have a good laugh. A crisis can heighten awareness and increase your appreciation of what is around you. By maintaining as normal a life as possible you are also creating a framework for coping with life should cancer be diagnosed.

Remember … There is life after diagnosis!

Live all you can; it's a mistake not to.

Henry James (1843–1916)

Section 2 Diagnosis

'I Have It!'

Choice 7

On Hearing The Big 'C'

Ill news is wing'd with fate, and flies apace.

John Dryden (1631–1700)

Hearing that you have cancer can be a terrifying experience. It may be completely unexpected and come like a bolt from the blue. You might have been undergoing routine surgery or tests. Very occasionally lumps which are thought to be harmless turn out to be cancerous. Perhaps you had not been told that you might have cancer. Even if you are partly prepared you may still be stunned.

'You have a tumour and we need to operate quickly. I'd like to book you in for this Monday.' It was Wednesday. I started to feel scared. Everything was happening so fast. I felt I was on a roller coaster. At this point I was obviously in shock. Thankfully my consultant understood and arranged for me to see him on Friday with my partner so that he could fully explain the situation. — Jo

Ironically, this was the first appointment for which my manager refused to give me time off. I felt a bit sick; guilty because I wasn't there even though in a million years how could you know what was going to happen? — Simon

When you are in shock it is hard to hear what is being said. It feels like all you can see in front of you is the word 'cancer'.

- If you think there is any chance of a diagnosis of cancer, take someone with you to the appointment. The other person will not be able to take away your fear but he or she can care for you when you are at your most vulnerable. A companion is also more likely to be able to listen to what the consultant is saying, while your mind is still reeling from the shock. It is a good idea to take a notebook and write down what the consultant tells you or even take a tape recorder so that you can listen again when you feel calmer.

It was terribly important that I was at all consultations – if people are anxious and worried they don't take things in. We could discuss what we were told later and talk about what things meant. I wanted to know what was going on and what Vicki was being told so that I would know the situation for myself. When something terrible happens to a loved one you want to know exactly. I remember asking the consultant to take good care of her, as she was very precious to me. — Barry

🍂 People react very differently to this situation. You might, for instance, feel totally paralysed for a moment or two. You may not believe the consultant. You may want to run out of the room. You may feel you are in some kind of surreal situation where nothing seems to make any sense. You may start giggling or laughing. You may not be able to speak for a while. All of these reactions are perfectly normal responses to shock. If you are on your own, ask for another appointment as soon as possible so that you can discuss the situation with someone to support you.

While I waited in the hospital corridor for a blood test, I recognised an acquaintance from work. 'How are you? What are you doing here?' he asked. 'I've just been told that I have cancer.' The voice does not seem to come from me; it is bleak and cold and matches the grey November day. — Vicki

🍂 You might want an opportunity to discuss your illness and treatment with a health care professional a few days later when you have had time to think about what you have been told. The consultant might suggest this to you or you can ask for an appointment yourself.

Having cancer diagnosed is frightening but at least you are no longer in limbo. You know what you are dealing with and can start taking control and make plans again.

Choice 8

Not Understanding Everything Doesn't Mean You're Stupid!

A s you try to come to terms with the diagnosis you may feel worried about asking what may seem to you like trivial or stupid questions. It can be difficult to digest medical information, particularly if you are feeling vulnerable. You may think that to the doctor you are just one more person with cancer but your world has just been turned upside down.

- It is important to understand your situation so don't be afraid to ask the consultant to repeat what has been said or to explain it in a different way. If you have someone with you, ask him or her to write down what the consultant is telling you. No question is too trivial. You can be sure that whatever questions are in your mind have been asked by many others before you.

Questions you might have:

- What stage has the cancer reached? Has it spread?

–   What happens now? Will I have to have further investigations? What treatment should I expect?

–   What is actually involved in surgery/radiotherapy/ chemotherapy?

–   What is the timescale for an accurate prognosis?

What does pre-cancer mean? That was the overriding question for me. Even though the consultant answered the question I still didn't know. He made it clear that until the ovary was removed he wouldn't be able to tell for sure. It felt like a no-win situation. — Simon

❧ Remember that each type of cancer affects people differently. It's not like breaking a bone for which there is usually a standard process of diagnosis and treatment. Unless you are an oncologist there is no reason why you should have any knowledge of cancer or of medical terms.

'You have a tumour and we need to operate quickly.' My mind raced; I knew it was serious but what does 'a tumour' mean? Is it the same thing as cancer? — Jo

❧ Find out only as much as you want to know at this time. Some people want to know everything; others choose not to. You might not, for instance, feel ready to ask about your prognosis. You will always have an opportunity to ask questions later on.

- If you think of questions you want to ask between appointments, make a list and take it with you to your next meeting with the medical practitioner.

- Try and frame the questions to get some of the answers you want.

> *I was so frightened about being given a poor prognosis that I decided to ask my second consultant what positives I had going for me. It worked; he told me that 89 per cent of his patients did very well. This gave me vast amounts of hope.* —Vicki

- You may feel you want to be included in the treatment process as part of a team rather than as someone at the bottom of a hierarchical structure. If so, you can discuss this with your doctor.

Choice 9

❧

Now Might Be The Time For Surfing And Reading

Reading is to the mind what exercise is to the body.

Richard Steele (1672–1729)

Now that you have a definite diagnosis, you will be clearer as to what you might want to know about your illness. You can get more information from books, information leaflets, the internet and other places.

❧ *Books.* There is a growing body of literature on cancer – its causes, its effects, its treatment. Reading can tell you how some people have coped with their illness and this can be comforting. You can feel very lonely when you have cancer and it is reassuring to know that you are not alone in what you are feeling. However, a bit of caution is sometimes needed. Some of the literature is contradictory. One book will recommend a particular diet or treatment plan; another will put the case for a different regime. Because cancer affects people differently, you may not find the perfect book for you. As we pointed out in Choice 4, reading about cancer can be frightening. At times what you read will inspire you into certainty that you will come through this ordeal; at other times your worst fears may be confirmed by what you are reading.

- *Information leaflets.* This is a good time to contact specialist organisations as they usually have booklets written in a down-to-earth way. They describe symptoms and the treatment of the particular form of cancer their organisation is concerned with. They are an excellent source of information. A list of some of these organisations can be found at the end of the book.

- *The internet.* If you have access to the internet you will find an overwhelming amount of information, some of which may well be conflicting. Take your time to work through it; it is useful to enlist the support of a friend who can help you determine what information is relevant and useful to you. A word of caution: anyone can put information on the internet. It is wise to check any medical facts given with your doctor.

- *Other people.* Some of your most useful information and support may come from those people who have had personal experience of your particular cancer. They understand what you might be going through and you don't have to keep explaining what is happening and how you are feeling. There are some organisations set up to provide people with such contacts. A list appears at the end of the book.

> *Women who had had breast cancer contacted me or offered to speak to me. I was grateful that total strangers who had been through the same experience reached out to me. It was a remarkable network and I hoped that my courage would match theirs. — Vicki*

Choice 10

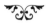

Second Opinion?

Why might you want a second opinion?

Because:

- It is your right.

- You may not yet have seen a cancer specialist.

- You may not feel particularly comfortable with the doctor you have seen.

- You may want to feel that you are getting the best available treatment.

- You may wish to have private treatment.

- You have heard of someone who has a particularly good reputation in this field.

> *I was angry with the consultant who gave me the diagnosis for the way in which he broke the news. Perhaps I would have hated anyone who told me that I had cancer but he left me feeling hopeless and defeated. I decided to seek a second opinion from a breast cancer specialist who agreed that a mastectomy was necessary. However, he assured me that I was going to be fine and backed up his statement with reasons. He gave me the strength to fight and I trusted what he said.*
>
> —Vicki

> *I didn't really think about getting another opinion, but someone asked me, 'If you were buying a second-hand car would you buy the first one someone tried to sell you?' That made me think and the cancer specialist from whom I sought a second opinion recommended further tests and transferred me to his care at a specialist cancer centre.* —Jo

What is against a second opinion?

- You may be confused if the two consultants disagree about the treatment you need.

- You have to go through the ordeal of seeing a consultant again.

৵ If you are hoping for good news you may be disappointed if the diagnosis is the same.

> *Vicki went to another consultant for a second opinion. He had a totally different approach in giving his opinion and long-term views of recovery. He gave both of us confidence in the way he dealt with each of us. He had a reassuring manner and a professional attitude. It was reassuring when he told us his statistics as these were particularly good.* — Barry

If you are thinking of asking for a second medical opinion you need to go through your GP. Of course, the choice is up to you, but we do feel that it is very important to see a cancer specialist. Although all consultants deal with cancer, the statistics suggest that patients do better with a consultant who specialises in a particular cancer and so is dealing with it all the time.

> *I received my diagnosis in the morning. I had pre-arranged to see my GP that afternoon in case the news was bad as I had read an article on breast cancer which said that it was vital to see a breast cancer specialist and one had been recommended to me who sounded really good. I felt secure knowing that I had that appointment booked.* — Vicki

Choice 11

Let Yourself Feel What You Feel

Below the surface-stream, shallow and light,
Of what we say we feel – below the stream,
As light, of what we think we feel – there flows
With noiseless current strong, obscure and deep,
The central stream of what we feel indeed.

Matthew Arnold (1822–1865)

Once it has been diagnosed that you have something like cancer your priorities change instantly. All the things you were worrying about can suddenly seem very trivial indeed. In fact you can find it difficult to believe that you worried about them at all. All that matters now is your life.

I felt I needed to strip away all the things that weren't essential like social activities and general day-to-day concerns. These were all put on a back burner. Normal problems became somewhat over-shadowed. Even so, missing the Arsenal v Manchester United game was difficult. However, my loyalty to Jo was paid back by the consultant, who being another Arsenal fan, rescheduled the op until after the FA cup final! — Simon

---

❧❀❧

How does this make you feel?

❧ There really is not a right way to feel about having cancer. You will probably be very frightened at first, worried that the cancer might have spread. At times you will just not believe this is happening to you.

❧ You might experience some surprising feelings. You may, for instance, feel extreme anger or bitterness at the unfairness of what is happening. 'Why me? Why should this be happening to me?' You might feel guilty, thinking that you have somehow brought the illness on yourself. You may feel that you are letting down those who are close to you as your illness is distressing for them.

I tortured myself wondering how long the lump had been there. I am an intelligent woman yet did not examine my breasts regularly. I was racked with guilt; if this was cancer and it had spread then my irresponsibility would cause those who loved me even more pain. — Vicki

❧ You may find you get headaches or other pains as a result of tension. It is easy to get into a panic state, thinking it is a new tumour. Don't let the panic overwhelm you; contact your GP or cancer support nurse to talk it out.

❧ Let yourself feel what you feel. Think of yourself as on a journey to a territory that is unknown. Sometimes the terrain will be easy to travel through – at other times the journey will be arduous and tiring. Do whatever you can to make the journey as easy as possible. When you feel tired, rest. If you feel angry find a safe way to express that anger. Punching a cushion or shouting at the wall can be amazingly therapeutic. Talk about your fears to a sympathetic person; often fear does diminish when it is put into words.

In spite of the fear, as the days went by I became aware that breast cancer was also changing my life in positive ways. I became much more open with family and friends and they with me; we cried and hugged together. —Vicki

Be willing to take life on trust and be proud of yourself for how you are succeeding. Just keeping going is an achievement at a time like this.

Choice 12

❦

When All Else Fails Try Scream Therapy!

People cope with anxiety in different ways and you will find your own way of managing your worry and fear. In Choice 2 we suggested some things that might help you to feel better while you were waiting to know what the situation was. Here are some of the coping mechanisms that worked for us once we knew we had cancer:

- ❦ Keep a diary. Things can seem less frightening when they are written down. You can confide to your diary those fears and worries which you don't want to tell anyone. Your journal will become your own personal record of this part of your life.

- ❦ Write exactly what you are feeling at a particular moment, however incoherent or irrational. No-one else need see this and you can tear it up later if you wish. You may be surprised at how therapeutic it can be to get your thoughts out onto paper.

- ❦ Make two lists. One list will be of all the things that

you have positively going for you; the other will be of your innermost fears. You will find that the positives outweigh the fears and this will be in your favour in your journey through cancer.

🐦 Take a trip into the past. Visit places where you used to live; where you were happy. Tell yourself that you will reach those places again. It is still possible to make your dreams come true, whether they are big or small.

🐦 Choose to be with the people in whose company you feel most relaxed.

Talking to friends and family was very important for Vicki. This helped me too. At the same time I could help friends and family as I had genuine confidence in the outcome. If Vicki had not talked to people we would both have been more isolated and I would have felt more responsible. — Barry

🐦 It's a good idea to be with people who are busy; getting involved with activity helps you to think about something other than your illness.

🐦 As well as seeking company, also allow yourself time on your own if the company of others becomes a strain.

❧ Find a place where you can give full vent to your feelings; where you can scream and shout if you wish.

The only time I really let go my feelings was when I was alone in my car. I turned the music up to its loudest volume and just screamed; it's amazing how therapeutic that was. I remember telling a friend who also had cancer what I did and she said: 'Really! I thought I was the only one who did that!' — Jo

---

Choice 13

Sometimes You'll Feel Up; Sometimes You'll Feel Down

A whirlwind does not last a whole morning.
A downpour of rain does not last a whole day.

Lao Tzu c. 700BC

We have already made the point that you will probably experience a range of feelings, some of which may well be unexpected and frightening.

This choice is about realising that you will have bad days and good days. The fear when we have a bad day is that there will never be a good day again.

🐦 If you are having a bad day, tell yourself that this is just a bad day, and that it will be followed by a good day. You may feel like a yo-yo as you go up and down and this can be unsettling if you are not used to mood swings. However, if you allow yourself to feel down and stay with those feelings, it is sometimes easier to move up again.

◦ It is impossible to be positive all the time. When you feel low let yourself weep and allow the tears to wash over you. This is a way of relieving tension.

The days passed in a kind of blur, with lots of tears. — Jo

◦ It is quite normal to feel as if you are being unpredictable and out of control; some days you may feel like hiding from the world because you feel so scared and tired; other times you will feel really positive and want to be with people.

◦ At times you may be calm and accepting and be able to carry on doing normal tasks. At other times the knowledge that you have cancer may overwhelm you. It may feel like being in a battle. The enemy is cancer and sometimes you feel that you will beat this enemy; other times you are not so sure. It can be a real struggle to try and be positive all the time when you do not know what you are fighting. However, with knowledge you will find out what you are up against and what hurdles you need to overcome. Victory cannot be guaranteed but being positive and in victory mode is a good place to be.

During the early days, as the family's optimist, I tried to sound hopeful and reassuring. Inwardly, I felt uncertain, scared and distracted. At times I remember thinking: 'If this is how I feel, how on earth does Mum feel?' — Laura

Choice 14

Who Needs To Know?

Those closest to you may already know the situation but now that things are more certain you need to think about whether there are any others whom you want to inform or who ought to know. Telling people can be very hard. Make it as easy as possible on yourself.

> *My thoughts were racing again. How was I going to tell my partner, mum and dad, sister, Nan? The list was endless. 'I'll remain calm,' I decided. 'Hello, darling, how did it go?' said Simon in such a cheerful voice. 'Not too good,' I replied through my tears – so much for remaining calm. —Jo*

❧ It is inevitable that those people close to you will be upset by your news and this knowledge can make it very hard for you to tell them. If at all possible, try to do it at a time when they are not alone and can be supported by others.

> *When Jo telephoned me with the news I was stunned and struck dumb – something hitherto unknown to me! —Anne*

I was three months pregnant when I first heard that Mum had breast cancer. I was teaching at school on a Friday and got the news during my lunch break. My initial feelings were of shock and disbelief because until then I kept hoping that she could not really have breast cancer. I remember being comforted by members of staff to whom I was close as I started to cry, although it was as if nothing they said was of any use or made me feel better at this time. —Jillian

'Surely people get cancer in other *families' was one of my first thoughts. I felt very possessive and very ignorant about what practical help I could offer. I didn't know anything.* —Cyril

Jo's diagnosis coincided with my finding out that I was pregnant. I wanted to tell her that I was pregnant but was worried about how she would feel, given the implications of her diagnosis for her future fertility. I also knew that I couldn't possibly not *tell her.*

Jo took the news of my pregnancy really well – she was honest about how she felt and I managed to say that I felt awkward telling her my news. We realised that the timing of the events was really ironic and we even managed to laugh about it but we also had a good chat about how we both felt.

—Laura

🕊 Create a 'telephone tree' by asking each person you tell to let others know. This means you don't have to keep repeating yourself and it also helps others to feel they are doing something practical to help you.

🕊 As people get to know they will probably want to contact you. This can be tiring particularly if several people telephone on the same day. If possible, get someone else to take your phone calls, or put on your answerphone so that you can speak to people when you feel up to it.

🕊 It is likely that your general practitioner referred you for tests. You may find it helpful to return to your GP so that you can discuss your diagnosis. Your GP practice can be a source of good support during the process of your treatment and will certainly be able to give you information about support available directly from them or from the community health services.

What might be reasons for not telling people?

The fact that people around us knew what was going on has been very helpful to us. However, everyone's situation is different and you may have good reasons for not telling. For instance:

❧ There may be people who would be so upset that they would not be able to cope.

❧ It can cause problems if you are in a leadership role or if there are a lot of people depending on you.

❧ You may worry about being the subject of conversation or being out of control of the information people have about you.

What about young children?

It is particularly distressing and worrying if there are young children who are going to be affected by what is happening. Obviously you will want to be careful about what they are told because you won't want to frighten them unnecessarily. Whether you tell them or not is a decision you will have to make. Remember, though, that even very young children have an almost uncanny way of picking up the atmosphere and that it can be more frightening for them to know there is a secret but not know what it is, than to have some information.

❧ If you are worried about how to tell any children involved, it is worth seeking advice from a counsellor, social worker, your GP, teachers or any other professional who has experience of this kind of situation.

◦➤ A guiding principle is to answer any questions and don't tell the children more than they need to know at any particular time.

◦➤ There are some very good children's books which deal with this kind of situation and which might help you to introduce the subject.

◦➤ If and when you do choose to speak to the children, try to choose a time when they are at their most relaxed.

I notice that it is when I am bathing my grand-daughter, Sarah, that she confides her thoughts to me. — Vicki

Choice 15

Other People's Reactions

Finding out that you have cancer is distressing enough. You are trying to manage your fears and worries and carry on with whatever needs to be done. You may find, however, that you are not only trying to deal with your own reactions but those of the people around you as well. Just as you are experiencing a range of feelings, those close to you will be coping with their own shock, sadness, fear and worry for you. How others manage these feelings can cause you surprise. Some people will find just the right thing to say or do which makes you feel supported; others just can't seem to handle the situation.

I knew the news was not good when I realised that Jo was crying. My first thought was, 'This is wrong; it should be me.' I didn't know what to say at first; all I could do was give her a big hug. — Sheila

I knew the news would be bad as Jo did not ring from the hospital but just appeared on the doorstep crying. I was very conscious that my usual calm approach counted for nothing when my own flesh and blood is concerned. I could not prevent

my natural reaction of both horror and foreboding from showing on my face. Intellectually I knew this was not helpful but emotionally it was all I could do at the time. — Cyril

When Jo told me her news, I thought, 'How could this be? She is the same age as my daughters. What can I say?' Trite phrases were out of the question! — Anne

As the days passed before Mum had her mastectomy, I was filled with a range of emotions. I was angry and shed a great many tears. — Jillian

I didn't cry for ages and then only on my own. — Simon

You are bound to experience a range of reactions from the people you tell.

❧ Some people just seem to find a way to make you feel better.

Words, both expected and unexpected, helped. I rang a work acquaintance to cancel a meeting and started by saying: 'I have some bad news.' Before ending the conversation he told me that he was thrilled that I was going to be all right. 'I expected to hear that you are terminally ill; instead you say you are going to be fine.' It was a wonderful response when I had got used to receiving commiseration. — Vicki

❧ You may be surprised, even hurt, by some people's reactions to your news. Some people can't seem to mention the word 'cancer'; others can't talk about anything else. Some people will try to jolly you along as if by making you feel better they can feel better themselves.

> *I was disappointed by some people's reactions and heartened by the unexpected kindness and sympathy of others.* — Simon

❧ Sometimes a gesture is as helpful as words.

> *Friends bought me a bonsai tree kit – 'So you can watch the tree grow next year'. My hairdresser, without telling me, made me an appointment for Christmas Eve.* —Vicki

❧ Some people feel too uncomfortable to know how to communicate. It can be very hurtful when people from whom you expect support seem to avoid you. Very often this is because the person is afraid of saying or doing the wrong thing. If someone who is important to you is apparently avoiding you, you could take the initiative just to say that you want to be in contact. Maybe someone is going through a traumatic time and either doesn't want to burden you with it or just doesn't have the resources to help you. So the apparent avoidance isn't really personal.

❧ Decide what kind of support would help you most and then seek contact with those people who can give you that support. Think about creating a network rather than relying on one or two people. Support can have many facets and it is unfair to expect one person to be able to meet all your needs. The following are some of the needs you might identify:

— Someone with whom you can cry

— Someone with whom you can laugh

— Someone who will share you greatest fears

— Someone who sees the bright side

— Someone who can be practical

— Someone with whom you can be quiet

— Someone who can distract you

— Someone who is a reliable source of information.

Make your own list and write the names of people who you think would fill the need. If there are any gaps, maybe you can think about how to fill them.

Choice 16

You Are Not Alone

*Down in their hearts, wise men know this truth:
the only way to help yourself is to help others.*

Elbert Hubbard (1859–1915)

This choice is about finding support outside your circle of friends and relations. Some of the organisations set up to help cancer sufferers have organised a network of support groups (see list at end of book). These are groups of people who have or have had cancer; they meet regularly to share their thoughts and feelings and give each other support, information and advice. There are many different kinds of groups:

- The groups can either be self-programming or run by a leader who manages the discussion.

- Some groups welcome relatives or carers.

- They can be very informal, perhaps meeting in someone's house or, more formally, meeting in a hospital or on council premises.

❧ Some groups are workplace-based.

❧ There are groups specially organised for people with a particular kind of cancer; others are more general.

❧ Whether you decide to contact a group just now is up to you. Some people find them most helpful; others do not.

> *Support groups are not my sort of thing. I especially did not want to talk to someone who had cancer.* — Simon

Groups can help in a number of ways:

❧ Meeting people who are going through the same kind of experience as you often allows you to talk freely and feel understood.

❧ People may have very useful information and advice which can help you out in a practical way. You can see how other people are coping.

❧ It is always good to know you are not alone.

❧ Groups can be a safe place to let go of your emotions.

❧ The group meetings are not always full of gloom and doom. You could well find that you have a good laugh; somehow it is possible to see the funny side of some of the things which happen and sometimes the atmosphere can be very light-hearted.

Emotionally I felt that I needed to be with people who were going through the same experience as I was. It made me realise that I wasn't on my own. — Jo

Choice 17

Can A Counsellor Help?

'The time has come,' the Walrus said,
'To talk of many things.'

Lewis Carroll (1832–1898)

We all have our own way of facing our problems. Some of us like to go it alone, managing as well as we can. At other times we may turn to friends and family. At a time like this in your life you will be relying to a great extent on professional helpers such as doctors, social workers, nurses and so on. Counsellors and therapists are among those who are available to help us through the problems of living. They use their skill and knowledge to help us deepen our understanding and control of the emotional aspects of our situation. Through a process of regular meeting and talking they work to help us make decisions and manage our lives.

If you are used to working with a counsellor you will be familiar with the particular help that counsellors can give. If you have never been to a counsellor but are considering the possibility, here is some information that might help you decide.

How does counselling work?

When you go to a doctor or other medical expert you expect him or her to diagnose, advise, instruct, interpret and direct you. You are more or less the passive partner receiving guidance from the expert. Going to a counsellor is a very different experience. Counsellors aim to help you through building up a special relationship based on mutual trust and respect. They use their skills and knowledge to help you live your life as happily and resourcefully as possible. The advantage of such helpers is that they have no vested interest in how you decide to run your life. The therapy they offer is an opportunity to evaluate yourself and your life objectively so that you can make wise and appropriate decisions about the future.

Sessions usually take place in a consulting room which might be in the therapist's home, a health centre, GP practice or some other appropriate location. Counselling sessions are usually around an hour in length, perhaps once a week. Most counsellors will negotiate the frequency of sessions depending on circumstances.

When you are with the counsellor you will spend most of your time together talking but it won't be like the conversations you are used to. Because the counsellor is trying to understand you as much as possible, he or she will spend most of the time listening while you talk. It won't matter how long it takes you; you will find that there are times when you don't really know what to say or you might want to think about something before you speak. When the counsellor joins in the conversation it will often be to reflect back what he or she has understood you to be saying and how you might be feeling. Sometimes he or she might be right and sometimes wrong and you will have the chance to clarify your thoughts if you want to.

The counsellor is more interested in understanding and accepting you than in judging whether you are right or wrong, silly or sensible, good or bad. You might find it odd that the counsellor does not try to 'make you feel better' if you are feeling down; the focus will be on helping you understand and face your feelings. The reasoning behind this is that distressing feelings don't disappear if we ignore them – they may fade for a while but are likely to come up again and again. Counsellors believe that discharging such stored-up emotions can be a healing process, leaving more energy free for the business of everyday living.

It was a relief to have the chance to honestly say how I was feeling because I tended to put on different faces for different people. The counsellor gave me the opportunity to stop my thoughts racing and not give myself such a hard time. —Jo

~ ❧ ~

Having an illness like cancer can bring up problems from the past that you thought had long been dealt with. Perhaps there is some 'unfinished business' that you still feel guilty about; maybe old feelings of helplessness overwhelm you; maybe memories of deaths or illnesses you have faced in your family come back to haunt you. Counselling can help you understand and manage these emotional processes.

> *Counselling did help. It was nice to talk to someone with no agenda.* — Simon

To find a counsellor, contact:

- a national association for counselling, e.g. British Association for Counselling

- your general practitioner

- your hospital department

- your place of employment

- one of the organisations set up to help people with cancer.

Choice 18

When Panic Rules!

I have a faint cold fear thrills through my veins,
That almost freezes up the heat of life.

William Shakespeare (1564–1616)
ROMEO AND JULIET

However well you are managing this difficult period in your life there are bound to be times when it just all seems too much and your fears and anxieties take over. Below are some of the ways you can help yourself get over these times.

Relaxed breathing

Our nervous system has a two-part response to stress; our first automatic response triggers what is usually known as the 'flight/fight' response. This means that you tend to breathe more quickly and more shallowly as your body produces more energy for you to deal with the threat. These reactions are brought into play by the sympathetic nervous system. However, we also have a parasympathetic system that can reduce the level of arousal and calm us down. It is this system that returns our heart rate and breathing to previous levels; redistributes blood back to the digestive system; lowers blood pressure and so on. Obviously if we can activate this system when we are under a lot of stress, we will feel much calmer. Controlling your breathing is one of the ways of doing this.

To bring the calming parasympathetic system into play, breathe more slowly and deeply. The temptation when we are anxious is to breathe in and then hold the breath. So concentrate on breathing out rather than breathing in.

Be relaxed
There are lots of different methods of relaxation. Learning a technique is a good way of taking control of your anxiety. Developing and using the skill of relaxation will take some time. However, regular relaxation will improve your ability to deal with your most anxious moments. The following very simple technique is called 'Counting Relaxation'. It involves counting down from ten to zero. The brief time needed to count backwards can break the spiral of anxiety and tension. The simplest way of doing this is to focus on your breathing while counting. Each time you breathe out say the next number. You could tape this script or get a friend to read it over for you.

Count backwards from ten to zero. Silently say each number as you breathe out. As you count you will feel more and more relaxed. When you reach zero you will be completely relaxed.

Ten ... feel the tension drain way; nine ... relax more deeply; eight ... more and more relaxed; seven ... deeper and deeper; six ... let yourself feel calm and relaxed; five ... as the tension drains away your body feels limp and heavy; four ... more and more relaxed; three ... deeper and deeper; two ... very relaxed now; one ... you're feeling calm and in control; zero ... absolutely relaxed.

Keep breathing slowly and deeply and let yourself drift into a feeling of calm and safety. Try to contact a feeling of inner peace and be aware of this feeling so that you can bring it to mind when you choose.

Now count from one to three; say each number to yourself and take a deep breath with each one. One ... relaxed but more alert; two ... still relaxed but wide awake; three ... eyes open, feeling refreshed. Keep the feeling of relaxation and calm with you as you move into whatever you are going to do next.

Vicki lent me a relaxation tape because I was finding it difficult to sleep. It is something that I had never done before. We got ourselves ready for bed, put on the tape and slowly for the first time in ages I felt myself really relax. I could even hear Simon snore although he says I was the first to go off. Just when

> *I had completely relaxed, this lovely quiet voice I was listening to became sharper and loud … 'Time to get up now!' We both woke up with a start – Vicki forgot to tell us it was a tape for day-time listening!* — Jo

Movies of the mind

You are probably already familiar with the way thoughts and images can be upsetting and add to feelings of fear and anxiety. However, visualisation can be a positive force for relieving stress and is often used together with relaxation as a very good way of calming down.

The basic technique is to form a clear image of a pleasant scene connecting with each of the five senses; e.g. sight: 'see the sparkle of the sun on the water'; smell: 'smell the scent of the flowers'; taste: 'taste the salt from the sea on your lips'; touch: 'feel the smoothness of the rock-face'; sound: 'hear the waves breaking on the shore'. Start with basic relaxation and breathing and create the picture in your mind.

> *I felt very tense and a friend suggested I thought of a place where I'd been really happy and encouraged me to create the image in my mind. It helped me relax my muscles and I felt less tense. I can still see the scene in my mind.* — Vicki

꽃

Meditation

Meditation is a way of relaxing your mind and focusing your energy. There isn't really a right way to meditate; there are many approaches and you may need to try several before you find one that suits you. Here is an example:

Find a place in which you can sit comfortably and without interruptions. There is no need to sit in a special position. Just make sure you are well supported and comfortable. You might want to set a timer so that you don't have to worry about when to finish. Fifteen to twenty minutes is a reasonable period to start with.

Breathe slowly and deeply and create an image in your mind of an object which has some meaning for you: a candle, a star, a vase, for example. Hold this image in your mind. You will find that at first your mind wanders and you start thinking of other things. When that happens, gently bring your mind back to the image.

There is in stillness oft a magic power
To calm the breast when struggling passions lower;
Touched by its influence, in the soul arise
Diviner feelings, kindred with the skies.

John Henry Newman (1801–1890)

Choice 19

Being Afraid You Are Going To Die Doesn't Mean You Can't Live Now!

Tomorrow I shall live, the fool does say;
Today itself's too late; the wise lived yesterday.

Martial (43–104)

This is a time in your life when you should indulge yourself. You will be very conscious of your body and what is going on in it. But we are more than a mind and body machine. Our spirit and feelings also need a lot of attention at times like this. These choices are all about how you can make sure your spirit is in as good a state as possible. Here are some things that have helped us:

- Massage is one of the oldest therapies around. However, there is some controversy as to whether it is an advisable therapy for people living with cancer. You will need to check with your medical practitioner whether it is safe for you to have a massage treatment. A study undertaken by Patricia McNamara (Co-ordinator 1990–93, Wandsworth Cancer Support Centre) and published in 1994 came to the conclusion that gentle massage by a skilled practitioner can be extremely helpful as an antidote to shock, panic or stress. The kind of massage that is enjoyable, calming, soothing and relaxing, making no demands on the person's body or mind, is potentially very therapeutic.

> *I did find massage treatment very soothing. It cut me off from a painful world, undid my knots; I could feel my body ease.* — Vicki

- Buy really nice underwear to take to hospital.

- Have a good haircut.

- Buy or borrow a personal radio/stereo to help you pass any sleepless nights and take into hospital with you.

- Try not to sit at home and brood; take daytrips to interesting places or go for walks.

- Take hot bubble baths. There is a great range of oils, herbs or lotions to choose from. Light candles to create a soothing atmosphere.

🐦 Give yourself food treats. Indulge in whatever takes your fancy. If you like chocolate, eat chocolate!

🐦 Look after a pet. Dogs and cats can be very calming and comforting.

🐦 Movement structures like Yoga and Tai Chi can be very calming and can also help to keep your body exercised.

Let the soul be joyful in the present, disdaining anxiety for the future and tempering bitter things with a serene smile.

Horace (65–8 BC)

Section 3 Treatment

'I'm Going Through It'

Choice 20

❦

'C' Stands For More Than Cancer

This section covers the time when you are going through treatment for your cancer. For many people it is a time of apprehension. While you are waiting for the treatment to begin, it is tempting to start recalling all the stories you might have heard about its effects. It is true that some treatments can be more unpleasant and exhausting than others.

> *Mum never really seemed ill immediately after the operation or during the following weeks' radiotherapy. I remember admiring her strength and wondering whether I'd have the same ability to cope if I ever had to go through this.* — Laura

> *When I saw Jo after one operation I just wanted to take out all the tubes and take her home.* — Simon

The 'C' word we want to emphasise at this point is Control, because this is something you may feel you lack! This is a time when other people seem to be making all the decisions: you may be receiving conflicting advice; you are given a timetable of treatments; your body feels like it is the property of the medical staff; you may feel you are losing your personal privacy; maybe other people are taking over things which you are accustomed to organising yourself. Feeling out of control can increase your feelings of helplessness and weakness. Of course you are reliant on your medical practitioners to a very great extent but there are still ways in which you can remain as much as possible in control of your situation.

- Be well informed. Ask as much as you want to about the treatment you are to receive. The things you need to know include:

  - What is the treatment intended to do?

  - How often will I need to have it?

  - How long will each treatment session take?

  - Where will it take place?

  - What kind of preparation would help me through the treatment sessions?

  - What are the possible side effects?

  - How can I best manage these?

  - Are there any ways in which I can lessen the side effects?

–   Are there things I can and cannot do during and after treatments?

–   Should I have someone with me while I attend sessions?

–   If I find that a particular drug I have been prescribed produces unpleasant side-effects, is there is an alternative?

You may be able to think of other questions which are important for you. Do not be afraid to ask them!

Nothing questioneth; nothing learneth.

Thomas Fuller (1606–1661)

❧ You are also more likely to feel in control if you understand all the options available to you. There may, for instance, be a number of different treatments for your condition; there may be a choice of hospitals or consultants and so on. Knowing your options can give you the opportunity of making choices. You can discuss options with your medical advisers, with other people who have had their own experience, with the advisers attached to the various organisations in our list at the end of the book, and with anyone else whose opinion you value and respect. Making an informed choice will help you feel more in control of things.

- We would recommend getting a second opinion from a cancer consultant if you have not already done so.

- We have already several times acknowledged that you are bound at times to feel afraid, depressed or angry. These feelings can leave you feeling drained and powerless. It can seem like these emotions are in control of you, rather than you in control of them. We have already suggested some ways of controlling these feelings so that they don't take you over completely. However, there may be times when the best thing to do is to accept how you feel at the moment rather than exhaust yourself even further by fighting the feelings.

Choice 21

The World Of Hospital

Yn ou will probably already be aware that there are several approaches to the treatment of cancer. Orthodox treatments include surgery, radiotherapy, chemotherapy and hormone therapy. There are also alternative therapies which include diet, vitamin and mineral supplements, detoxification, herbalism, homeopathy, acupuncture, relaxation, visualisation and spiritual healing. These can also be called 'complementary' therapies because they can be used alongside the orthodox treatments. We have a number of ideas that may help you through some of the orthodox treatments, particularly if they entail a stay in hospital.

If cancer is suspected or has been diagnosed, surgery is likely to be recommended. Some reasons for surgery are:

- To remove the tumour, surrounding tissues and the part affected by the disease

- To do a biopsy – removing a tissue so that its cells can be examined under a microscope. A biopsy may be undertaken if cancer is suspected.

Having surgery can be frightening because you don't know what the results might be. It can feel like stepping into an abyss and you need to find a foothold. At the same time you are moving forward, continuing your cancer journey in order to reach a place where you can feel safe.

> *I can't believe I'll lose my left breast tomorrow. I don't care as long as I live.* — Vicki

❧ Make a list of things to take with you into hospital. Your list might include:

– Boiled sweets

– Fruit juice

– Magazines, books

– Pen and notepad for consultant visits

– Walkman, tapes and CDs

– Change for the pay phone and newspaper trolley

– Earplugs

– Nice soap, face and hand cream.

And lots of treats!

If you are worried about how your household will run while you are away do anything that will help to put your mind at rest.

～ Make sure your partner knows how to work the washing machine and so on.

～ List any household bills that might be coming in so that things can just be kept ticking over.

～ Or do nothing and let everyone else get on with it!

When I had my first operation, I was scared because I had no idea of procedure. I arrived at seven in the morning as requested. At one o'clock the anaesthetist said there might not be a bed for me. Then suddenly I was on my way to theatre. I remember I had a pounding headache. —Jo

Admission to hospital can be the day before or the actual morning of the operation. You will probably be seen by an anaesthetist, have blood taken, be weighed and so on. Various members of the medical profession will probably ask you lots of questions about your medical history. You could think of writing out a kind of medical CV so that you can be sure of not forgetting anything. It's sometimes hard to remember details of all previous surgery, names of hospitals and dates, drugs you've been given, allergies, next of kin, any serious illnesses/conditions previous and present, name and address of your GP – to mention just a few of the questions you may be asked.

Anaesthetics can be scary if they are a new experience for

you. Different hospitals have different procedures. An anaesthetist will come and talk to you before the operation. You will probably be asked whether you have had anaesthetics before and how you reacted. If you have had a bad reaction make sure you tell the anaesthetist. There are often ways in which they can make changes so that you feel better when you are recovering. You might also want to ask the anaesthetist or nurse to explain the procedure for recovery from the operation. You are likely to be closely monitored for the period immediately following the operation. Your blood pressure and temperature will be taken frequently – perhaps as often as every five minutes.

You may be worried about suffering pain after surgery. Most pain can be contained by drugs and there are different ways of doing this. Your doctor should explain to you how pain will be relieved.

Waiting for results after surgery can be the most difficult time of all. It is bound to be a relief to know your operation is over but at the same time you are likely to feel vulnerable, possibly in pain and still in limbo until you are given the results. You cannot move forward until you know your prognosis. Check Choice 18 again for some ideas about coping with this time.

Each person's reaction to being in hospital is unique. It is like being in a different world. Some people are desperate to get home. Others feel protected, nurtured, safe, cut off into an unreal world. To some extent how you feel will be related to the kind of treatment you get in your particular hospital.

> *In the first hospital I was in, I was desperate to get home because everyone on the staff was so busy and I kept feeling I was a nuisance. In the second hospital I was so well looked after that I felt vulnerable about going home.* — Jo

At times you might surprise yourself at how cheerful and optimistic you feel; at others the fear and anxiety which is lurking underneath makes itself felt. Our advice is:

- Enjoy what you can enjoy when you can enjoy it. Visitors, for instance, can be a mixed blessing. Most hospitals offer very generous visiting hours but there may be times when you feel too tired to make conversation. Don't be afraid to let people know what you want. You might want to ask someone to read to you or just sit with you. Let people know if you have had enough of company for a while. Perhaps you could ask someone who is close to you to take some control of when people can come to see you and how long they should stay.

I felt I wanted to be at the hospital all the time because when I wasn't visiting Jo I was thinking and worrying about her. At least when I was there I felt I could somehow make her get better. I tried not to stay too long or do things which might make her tired but it was a hard time particularly when I felt she wasn't getting the standard of care I felt she should.

— Sheila

Unbidden guests are often welcomest when they are gone.

William Shakespeare (1564–1616)
HENRY V

- Don't be afraid to bother hospital staff. State your needs and don't hide your worries. If you feel you cannot do this yourself, ask someone to take up things on your behalf. It is so easy to feel passive and compliant when you are in hospital. It's a bit like being a child again – dressed in pyjamas and lying in bed! You can feel quite daunted at the idea of speaking to the nurses and doctors because they seem so busy and important.

- We suggested some questions you might want to ask about treatment. Here are some more questions that can help prepare you for hospital.

– Do you offer anything to help me if I feel anxious about the operation (often called 'pre-med.' which has a sedative effect)?

– I'm worried about being sick when I come round. Is there anything that would prevent this? (This is something to ask the anaesthetist.)

– How long will the operation take? It is quite a good idea to double the time you are told because operations can take longer than the forecast and that is incredibly worrying for anyone waiting for news.

– Will I have any tubes or a catheter attached? What will it feel like? For how long will I have them?

– When will the doctor visit me? (This question is important because you might want someone to be with you when the doctor comes.)

– Will I be able to go to the toilet on my own?

– Is radio/television/library, etc available? Do I have to pay for them?

❧ Take some things that will help you pass the time. As you recover and begin to feel better there will probably be spaces of time which you need to fill. So take books, a personal radio/ tape recorder and anything else you think will keep your mind busy. However, don't be surprised if you find it much more difficult to concentrate than you would normally.

🐦 Find out where the buzzer to summon a nurse is situated – and use it if necessary.

Types of treatment
Two of the well-known treatments for cancer are: radiotherapy and chemotherapy. These take place in hospital on an in- or out-patient basis or in your own home.

🐦 Radiotherapy can take place on a daily basis for several weeks or can be less frequent. Once again, being informed will help you understand what is happening so ask the questions on the list in Choice 20 you would like answered.

🐦 The treatment can feel frightening at first although it only takes a minute or two. It is not likely to be painful but you are normally in a room on your own with the machinery although, of course, you are being observed.

What I found most scary is that I was on my own, half-naked, with machinery whirring. I wanted to run away the first time. In order to try and control my fears I decided to while away the time counting. I did this each session to see if I reached the same number before the radiotherapy ended. Gradually I got into a routine and felt less nervous. —Vicki

❧ You will meet other patients while waiting for your radiotherapy. This can be very supportive. It can also be alarming if they are being treated for a recurrence of cancer.

I got so scared and sick inside listening to patients talking about recurrence. However, they all seemed so bright and positive and I realised that I, too, might be able to deal with a recurrence if it happened to me. —Vicki

❧ For some cancers, chemotherapy is the treatment of choice and this is the treatment which many people worry about. 'Chemo' affects each person differently. You may already have read about possible side-effects but this does not mean they will happen to you. The type of chemotherapy your doctor thinks you need may mean you temporarily lose your hair or your fertility can be affected. You could also feel nauseous or vomit although there are treatments to counteract these effects. Such concerns are best discussed with your doctor. The treatment can be given orally or intravenously (by injection). It can take place over anything from one to fourteen days; then there is usually a rest period for a few weeks. The length of the treatment depends on the type of cancer and how well it responds to drugs.

- Once again our advice is to arm yourself with as much knowledge as you want. Ask your doctor any questions that you have about the purpose and possible effects of the drugs you are to be given.

- If you don't feel too confident about asking your doctor, you will find that the helpline organisations set up all over the country (see list at end of book) will be able to give you information and advice. They may be able to put you in touch with someone who has had experience of the treatment you are facing.

Choice 22

Coming Home From Hospital

Who has not felt, how sadly sweet
The dream of home, the dream of home.

Thomas Moore (1779–1852)

It can be a huge relief when you are finally given a discharge date, but it can also feel scary to know that you will be away from the medical staff who have been looking after you. Here are some questions you might want to sort out regarding your discharge from hospital:

—   How will I get home? If someone is collecting me, where can he or she park?

—   Am I clear about any medication I will need when I return home?

—   Have I got clear instructions about what I will and won't be able to do once I return home? For instance, can I lift things, walk, run, swim, climb stairs and so on? If I can't do any of these, for how long will that last?

– What should I do if I feel unwell? Are there normal reactions I should be prepared for?

I was in a lot of pain and it was hard not knowing whether it was normal or not. The instructions I was given were quite vague and so I didn't know what it was safe for me to do. In hospital it seemed OK to depend on the medical staff but I found it difficult to depend on Simon and family for what seemed like silly little things, like help with getting up. —Jo

❧ Make sure before you leave hospital that you know what the arrangements are with regard to visits by a district nurse to check and change dressings if that is necessary. You are likely to feel more confident and secure if you know that someone will be keeping an eye on you once you are at home.

However much you may have been longing to get out of hospital, it can take some time to adjust to being at home again. You may find that you miss the routine and the support and companionship of other patients.

It was very strange coming home. There was my lovely familiar home but everything felt different. —Vicki

There is a lot for you to face once you are home, not least

yourself and your fears. Your feelings of vulnerability are unlikely to vanish overnight. A change of venue doesn't necessarily mean a change of thoughts. Hopefully the cancer has gone from your body but the fear may still be in your mind.

Even though your surroundings are familiar, at times you may feel you are in a strange new world. You will want to return to normality but progress may be slow. If you don't feel well, you are more likely to be low, weepy and even bad tempered. You may find it difficult to sleep and everything seems to be more frightening when you are lying awake at night. Relaxation can be a great help (see Choice 18).

I was delighted to have Vicki at home after the operation. I wanted to look after her to make sure that things went as smoothly as possible. I wanted things under my control and to deal with them as they cropped up, as quickly as possible. I was impressed with the way Vicki acted in being well and positive.
— Barry

Rest, don't overdo things, take good care of yourself, allow people to help you. You will feel better but you need to be patient because your progress is likely to be an up and down affair.

Being at home for such a long time was frustrating in some ways but I began to see there was a good side to it. People came to see me because I wasn't able to drive and I enjoyed spending time with them. I began to enjoy afternoon TV, and I'm still hooked on 'Dallas' repeats! — Jo

- If you are at all worried about your recovery contact your GP or the hospital to check whether everything is going according to expectation.

- You will probably find that your lifestyle will change when you are at home especially if you are used to being very active or going out to work.

When I was recovering from my operation, I went to see 'Carousel'. I identified with the song 'You'll never walk alone'. I had been through the storm of storms and come out on the other side. — Vicki

Choice 23

❧

Appearances Can Change

One of the big worries about cancer treatments is how your appearance can change. You can be scarred or your body shape can change. One of the effects of some chemotherapy, for instance, is that because the treatment affects all the cells, not just the cancerous ones, you can temporarily lose all your hair, even your eyebrows and body hair. Surgery can deprive you permanently of the part of your body that was affected. These losses can be very distressing and so we want to pay some attention to how you might approach this part of your cancer journey.

❧ Firstly, if you are worried about losing your hair, remember that no-one ever goes bald permanently from chemotherapy. Your hair will regrow when the chemo is completed and, in fact, the process can be quite an intriguing one because often the new hair is different. It may be a different colour; curly hair can grow back straight or straight hair can grow back curly.

❧ If you are facing hair loss it's quite a good idea to get into the habit of wearing a hairnet at night; and if you opt for a wig, under it during the day. This makes the loss less obvious. You could think about getting your hair cut into a very short style so that the loss is less traumatic. If you decide to get a wig, a synthetic one can be more comfortable to wear because it will be lighter than a natural one. You can indulge yourself in colourful scarves or hats – even make a fashion statement out of what you might worry is an unsightly state. And, of course, it is OK to be bald if you choose.

One of the things I read which really touched me was about a boy who had lost his hair as the result of chemotherapy. He was really worried about being bald when he returned to school. All of his classmates had their heads shaved so that when he arrived he was no different from anyone else. In a similar vein I also heard of someone whose whole family did a 'sponsored head shaving' for charity. These seemed great ways of making something positive out of something which could be so negative for the person involved. — Jo

- Another 'biggie' is the anxiety often surrounding the loss of a breast as a result of a mastectomy to treat breast cancer. Breasts are very connected to our sexuality and so for some women it can feel as if they somehow are no longer 'real' women without a breast. Some women are afraid that their partner's feelings towards them will be affected; some partners are afraid that their feelings will be affected when they actually see the physical effect of the operation.

> *I was aware that it was difficult for Vicki losing her breast. I was determined to show that I was not affected. Losing the breast had no great meaning for me at all and I wanted to make a fuss of the other breast. It was an anxious time for Vicki when she had to look at herself and when she had to see my reaction to her changed body. I was just relieved that the breast and cancer had been removed to stop it from creeping into the lymph glands and other parts of her body.* — Barry

> *I was prepared to pay any price for my survival and felt that losing a breast did not diminish me in any way. Nevertheless, when I faced my body for the first time the day that I left hospital I cried for my lost breast.* — Vicki

In spite of all we have written, the loss of a breast is often devastating for the woman involved. This is why breast reconstruction is now offered to most women who have had a mastectomy. It can be done in a number of ways and although it cannot replace the lost breast exactly it is very successful and many women are delighted with the result. You might feel like making contact with someone who has had this procedure and would be willing to talk about and show you the result.

◆ Another change with which you might have to contend is weight gain or loss. Some treatments have weight change as a side effect.

◆ If you are afraid or worried about the effects of changes in your body as a result of your treatment, talk to someone about it. These worries are very hard to cope with on your own. If you have a partner you may find it therapeutic to share your feelings. We have already mentioned the value of talking to a counsellor who will be willing and able to help you talk about your deep-seated fears and worries. Or you may prefer to talk to a friend whose views you trust or to someone who has been through a similar experience. You may feel that some of your worries are trivial or that others wouldn't understand them. Nothing about this experience of coping with cancer is trivial; your anxieties are natural. Although we can't make them disappear altogether we do feel that finding someone with whom to share them will make them less daunting.

There is nothing ugly; I never saw an ugly thing in my life; for let the form of an object be what it may, light, shade, and perspective will always make it beautiful.

John Constable (1776–1837)

Choice 24

Needing Help Is Not A Weakness

Are you the kind of person for whom it is important to be seen as strong, reliable and independent? If you are, one of the most upsetting aspects of being ill is that there are bound to be times when you don't feel so strong, when you are not able to do everything yourself. At these times, asking for and accepting the help of others is probably your best way forward but for many people this is not as easy as it sounds.

We have some suggestions for making it easier to ask for and accept the help that will make your life a bit easier during this time.

- First of all, do you think any of these statements are true?

  - I think that people should manage their difficulties themselves and not trouble other people with them.

  - To ask for help is a sign of weakness.

  - Other people will think you are selfish if you accept their help.

- When people ask if you want help, they don't really mean it.

- It is wrong to burden other people with your problems; they probably have enough of their own.

- The best way to manage a problem is to do it yourself.

- People won't think much of me if I can't seem to manage.

- If I accept someone's help, I'll lose my independence.

If you recognise any of these, think again! Are they really true? Each one sounds as if it is absolutely right, but actually very few things are absolutely right or absolutely wrong. Mostly, the truth lies somewhere in between extremes of belief. If you tie yourself into believing something is absolutely true, you leave yourself no room for any kind of change. If it were possible to replace these ideas with ones which gave you some room for movement you would find life a lot easier. 'I think that people should manage their difficulties themselves and not trouble other people with them,' could become 'Most of the time I like to manage things myself, but it's reasonable to ask others for help when I feel too ill or tired to do it on my own.' This belief allows you to ask for and accept help when you need it rather than struggling on your own to manage.

🖎 You might need to give yourself a 'talking-to' every now and again to acknowledge what has happened and to give yourself permission to be sensible and rest. Looking after yourself will aid your recovery more than pushing yourself to extremes.

Even though you may not be used to depending on others, needing help is not a weakness. In fact those close to you are likely to want to help you but may well be feeling helpless and unsure as to how best to do it.

It was really hard for me that Alisa lived abroad but she was one of the main people that I could be honest with about how I was feeling and one of the few people I cried openly with. — Jo

I was jealous of how everyone was supporting and helping Jo out; I felt helpless and powerless and that somehow I had let my sister down. I felt guilty because I lived so far away.
— Alisa

🖎 Reflect on how your time is structured at the moment. You need to make a list of all the things you are doing and then put them in order of priority. It might help to talk this over with someone who can be a little more objective than you. For instance, you might put 'keeping the house clean' near the top of your list – but that might not be the most important thing to keep going just now. After all, most houses don't fall down because they aren't cleaned!

If you are nervous about actually asking for help, the following ideas might help.

🐦 Be specific about what you want. 'Would you clean the bathroom?' is better than 'Could you help around the house?' 'It would help me if you would shop for the weekend meals' is better than 'Can you do the shopping?'

I was always pleased when Jo asked me to do something practical like looking after the dog for a while or going with her to the hospital. Although they were only small things, I did feel that I had some role that I could play. — Sheila

---

🐦 If you need something to be done by a certain time be clear about it. 'I would appreciate a lift to the hospital for my 2 o'clock appointment on Thursday; the appointment usually takes an hour' is better than 'Maybe you could give me a lift sometime.'

🐦 If someone asks you if he or she can be of any help,

think before you respond with 'No thanks, I can manage.' If there is something, say so; if not say thanks for the offer and ask if you can take a raincheck!

People must help each other; it is nature's law.

Jean de La Fontaine (1621–1696)

❧ There may be times when you don't want anyone around. It's perfectly OK to tell people this. If there is a regular time in the day when you like to rest, let people know. You can say something like: 'I'd love to see you; you just need to know that I'm usually asleep between 2 and 4 o'clock so it's a good idea to phone before you come so that you don't have a wasted journey.'

❧ There may be certain people you don't want to see perhaps because they are very negative or particularly tiring or for some other reason. This is obviously a little more difficult! However, this is a time to be looking after yourself so see if you can find a way to put them off. Maybe you can say something like: 'Thank you for your concern/interest/offer of help. I'd like to see you but I'm sure you understand that just at the moment I need to rest, so let me get in touch with you when I feel a bit stronger.'

❧ One of the frustrating problems you may have to contend with is that your mood might fluctuate much more than you are used to. One minute you may feel like crying and be full of despair; the next you feel positive and full of hope. It can be very difficult for other people to tune into your moods so the more you can say about how you are feeling at the moment the easier it is for them. There is nothing worse than someone trying to be upbeat and cheerful when all you want to do is cry on his or her shoulder for a while. The people close to you will want to be as helpful as possible but there will be times when they won't know just what you want. The more they understand about how you are feeling the better they will be able to help.

❧ If you have no support for practical help with, for example, cleaning or childcare, it is worth contacting your hospital social worker or local social services department to discuss the possibility of home support.

Choice 25

The World Of Work

*I like work; it fascinates me. I can sit and look at it
for hours, I love to keep it by me:
the idea of getting rid of it nearly breaks my heart.*

Jerome K. Jerome (1859–1927)

You may wonder whether to return to work while still undergoing treatment. It is helpful to keep a structure and lead as normal a life as possible while everything feels so uncertain. However, in returning to work you are entering a new phase and all new phases can make you feel vulnerable. You may feel fit enough now to return to work but it's natural to have some concerns.

Worries you might have:

- Will I be able to sustain a full day at work or will I be too tired to work well?

- Will I be able to concentrate fully or will I be too preoccupied with myself?

🍂 How will my colleagues react? How much should I talk to them about my condition? Will they feel burdened with my fears and feelings?

> *On hearing of Jo's cancer one of my first thoughts was, had I put her under pressure when she was working for me in a very busy agency? She worked very hard and was always ready, able and willing. Was the stress too much for her?* — Anne

> *Some colleagues just listened and quietly gave support. Others felt unable to face me although they worked in the caring environment of social services. They pretended that nothing had happened, that life was unchanged and I found myself colluding in that process.* — Vicki

If you do decide to return to work while still undergoing treatment it is important to think about all the implications and to discuss them with the appropriate people in your workplace. You may need to discuss how to arrange the time for your treatment sessions. You might think that it would be wise to negotiate a reduction in your hours for the time being or be helped in some other way. Most workplaces have a natural support system so you need to get to know it and use it fully.

However, sometimes things are not so easy.

While I realised I was fortunate with the support I got in my present job I know that if I were working elsewhere it would probably have been more difficult. — Jo

When going to work to explain what had been going on I took it for granted that I would get as much time and help as needed. In fact, what happened was that every obstacle was put in my way. When I applied for special leave I was told I probably wouldn't get it. Even when Jo was in hospital I was never allowed to leave early. In the end I was sent to occupational health as I took time off with stress. — Simon

❧ If you are self-employed, perhaps with a private practice, a number of questions may worry you. How soon you can return to work? How long will your clients wait for you? Will they remain loyal? Will you be able to give them the quality of service they expect? There are obviously no easy answers to these questions. If you have a local support network, do use it. Other professionals are very likely to be able and willing to help you. Think about whether there are any aspects of your work that could be delegated to someone else for a while. Administration, publicity, filing and so on are examples of matters that could be taken on by someone else. If you are able to afford it, you might employ someone or use an agency to take over these tasks while you are recovering your strength.

Choice 26

Priorities And Worries

Whatever your priorities in life were before, they are bound to change as a result of your illness. On a practical level, your treatment schedule will become a priority around which other things need to be fitted. You may want to give more thought to your diet, exercise and so on.

On the emotional level, too, things may have changed. Matters that seemed unimportant before can suddenly take on a new significance.

- Give yourself time to think about what is most important to you now. Talk with those close to you about any changes that would need to be made so that you can attend to what is most meaningful for you.

- Somewhere high on your list will be the challenge of maintaining your physical and emotional health as well as possible. You might be very unused to putting yourself first in this way but if ever there is a time to do it it's now! Things which you could think about include the following:

— When do you want to be with other people and when do you want time alone?

— Do you need to make time for resting?

— If you are in treatment how can you make it as easy as possible for yourself?

Try to give treatment days another focus. Going shopping, visiting galleries, going to the cinema, feeding the ducks in the park, visiting a place new to you are all possibilities.

After each radiotherapy session we tried to make a point of going out for lunch or visiting a place where we had not been before. I didn't know there were so many lovely places so near the hospital. —Vicki

A word of warning about worries!
Whatever worries you had before you developed cancer will probably have receded into the background while you have been coping with your illness. However, cancer doesn't make these worries go away and as you start to resume your normal life these other concerns, large and small, will re-emerge.

> *I was always irritated by all the papers on the kitchen table. When I was diagnosed with cancer I decided that such a trivial thing would never worry me again. I knew I was getting better when I became irritated with the untidy kitchen table once more.* —Vicki

It is difficult to see things clearly when you are feeling afraid or low so this may not be the best time to make life-changing decisions. If you feel that some decisions cannot wait then discuss what you want to do with someone whose judgement you trust.

> *I have had five weeks so far to recover from the last op. There are still so many questions buzzing around my head. Did I make the right decision to delay the hysterectomy? Have I endangered my life? Will the cancer come back? Should I put my body through a pregnancy? What is strange is that when I ask myself what it more important – living or being a mother – I struggle to find an honest answer because I know that if I had a child my answer would be different.* —Jo

This could be a good time to start thinking how you might handle worries differently in the future. If you have a stressful job, for instance, are there better ways of handling that stress? Maybe this is a good time to see a counsellor (see Choice 17) to help clarify your thoughts.

Priorities And Worries

❧

*The challenge is to learn to respond immediately
to whatever it is time for.*

Attributed to St. Benedict

Choice 27

Families Can Be Fragile

*All happy families resemble one another; every unhappy
family is unhappy in its own way.*

Tolstoy (1828–1910)
ANNA KARENINA

Each family has its own balance of relationships, rather
like those decorative mobiles which you can hang from
the ceiling. One member of the family becoming ill
changes that equilibrium just as increasing or decreasing
the weight of one of the elements of the mobile would
change its balance. Each member of the family deals with
the situation in his or her own way.

---

*It happened that I was in the bath when my sister telephoned
to tell me she had cancer. I just wanted to stay in there and
wash the sadness away.* —Alisa

---

*Mum phoned me at work to give me the results of her biopsy. As
soon as she told me I felt a rush of emotions – shock, worry, fear
and uncertainty. Everything had changed.* —Laura

> *I remember being comforted by colleagues to whom I was close as I started to cry but it was as if nothing they said was of any use or could make me feel better this time.* — Jillian

> *When Jo left us to go home, I made myself very busy round the house. I felt quite blank for a long time – just got on with the jobs I needed (or thought I needed) to do.* — Sheila

> *You learn it doesn't matter how you mentally prepare yourself. It's still such a shock. It was very hard to know what to say or do but just be there.* — Cyril

A close and supportive family can be a great source of strength and support.

- Allow yourself to take advantage of any help your family offers. Letting them help you is a way of helping them to feel less powerless.

- You might get the sense you are under scrutiny and this can make you feel defensive. Do what you have to do to get through.

However, some families are not so close. You may find that your illness actually strengthens your family, bringing people together. On the other hand, it may show up the cracks even more and you may need to protect yourself against the effects of whatever family conflicts exist. You may choose to try to resolve the problem yourself if you have the inclination and the energy. You may decide, though, that this is not the time for you to do anything about it. You could perhaps leave others to try to deal with the problem or just ignore it. You do, after all, have yourself to look after and that has to be your priority for now.

Choice 28

❧

Take Your Partner Along

*To be capable of steady friendship and lasting love
are the two greatest proofs, not only of goodness of heart,
but of strength of mind.*

William Hazlitt (1778–1830)

Watching someone you love suffer emotional and physical pain can almost be worse than suffering the pain yourself. Partners may feel helpless in that they cannot stop the cancer. However, they can be there for you, helping you cope with your own feelings.

> *I was anxious when Vicki moved on to radiotherapy. It was all new to me. Things had gone as well as expected and I hoped it would be successful. It was important that I was with Vicki when she went for treatment. I wanted to support her at all times.* — Barry

The various hospital procedures can be confusing and tiring for your partner. They often also have the added pressure of forcing you to wait around with little or no information about what is happening to you.

> *In the first hospital Jo was in, I was kept in the dark and seemed to be a nuisance to the staff. They didn't seem to know how worried I was. The second hospital very much included me in all the procedures. I was kept informed and treated with courtesy and respect.* — Simon

Partners need support too. They cannot be giving all the time and they have their own needs, practical and emotional, which require fulfilling.

> *I didn't crave emotional help although at times it was nice. My real needs were practical.* — Simon

> *Simon seemed to be so strong and it was an extra worry for me that he was not getting support. I really appreciated the people who asked how he was.* — Jo

> *I was not involved deeply with too many friends. I felt I had to cope in my own way although family and friends asked how I was coping and if they could make things easier for me. It was nice when a friend of Vicki sent me a card thanking me for helping Vicki. I had small anxieties. I was fairly new to London and worried about finding the hospital when Vicki was admitted for her operation and finding my way home in the dark.* — Barry

It is so easy to find yourself with feelings of guilt. Because you don't want to burden your partner and your partner doesn't want to add to your stresses, you might decide to hold back information from each other. This inevitably leads to poor communication and misunderstandings. Cracks can turn into crevices. The best thing, in the long run, is for each of you to be as open as you can about your feelings. This way, things are out in the open and you can face them together rather than battle on your own.

Partners have their own lives. Family and work commitments have to be maintained, for example. At the same time they need time for themselves and it can be as important for them to be able to talk to others about what they feel, as it is for you.

Partners do feel pain. This was a crisis in our relationship and I wondered how it would affect it. It was not as though we had been together 20 years. In a short relationship you are not sure how the other person will react. I was always anxious if Vicki wasn't well after she had cancer. It's easy to worry about a sore throat or any illness not connected with cancer. Every extra thing gives you anxiety. — Barry

Choice 29

❦

Friends And Neighbours

So far we have looked at how families and partners can be of great support, but of course not everyone has a close family or a partner. So a network of friends who are able to give comfort and support is also extremely important at times of crisis.

Throughout my pregnancy, which spanned several operations for Jo and a great deal of worry and uncertainty, I tried hard not to ignore the fact that I was pregnant but also tried not to go on about it. Jo had to cope with the physical and psychological effects of several operations and a lot of bad and uncertain news. We often talked about how she felt and I wished that I could do more to help than just be a voice and an ear down the phone line. — Laura

---

My friends suggested that we have a 'healing ritual' for Jo. We all lit a candle for her and sent positive energy. It made me feel much closer to her. — Alisa

---

When I first heard I thought, 'Why Jo?' but then I thought,

'Knowing Jo – she will cope.' There are times when I get upset but when I hear Jo's voice she is so hopeful, positive and strong.
— Breeda

When Jo first told me she had cancer I know I wanted to do anything to keep her alive. I couldn't do anything medically so I did things that were practical. I went round with videos during the day so she would have something and someone to get up for and 'put on her face' for. We cried over the videos and we laughed over us crying. It didn't matter whether we were laughing or crying as long as we were together. — Sandy

I think Jo and Simon have coped really well and I admire them immensely. I have spoken to Jo on many occasions through the good times and the bad and we have had many a heart-to-heart. All I can do is be there for them and listen. I think that is the key. — Sheena

I was around for Vicki. I was sympathetic but not necessarily reassuring. I helped Vicki to look at the implications. I could not tell her that she would be all right. I put my skills (as a psychologist) to use although it was more difficult than doing this professionally. I gave Vicki a relaxation tape I had made. What would I like to have done? Well, to have taken the cancer away. — Pauline

Vicki's cancer turned my life upside down. It was devastating. She was so important to me that it affected me badly. Vicki allowed me and others to be available to her. There was nothing that I couldn't talk about to her, even death. I was never pushed away. It was good to know that I was important to Vicki, that being there was what she wanted. I wanted to be around her. I was also grateful to Barry for all that he did. I should have liked to be able to tell Vicki that in five years she would be clear, that she would still be around. — Hélène

Being a friend is what you are. I listened to and empathised with Vicki. Over the years we had shared joys and sorrows. I should like to have been more around but I was teaching full-time. I should like to have been available during the day to share what Vicki was feeling. — Sylvia

I thought I had blanked everything out about Vicki's cancer, but recently a close friend collapsed and it made me remember how I had felt about Vicki. There were feelings of fear. I had a feeling of dread for Vicki as to what she was going to find out. There were also fears for myself and what was going to happen to me one day. I was an onlooker and felt helpless. I should have liked to have been there with Vicki whenever she needed me. — Sandra

Neighbours can be a further source of support. You may be friendly with them in which case you may choose to tell them about your cancer. Even if you do not know your neighbours well they may be surprisingly supportive if you choose to tell them what has happened to you.

> *When I was waiting to go into hospital I woke up feeling very low one day and dreaded going into work. On leaving home I had a chat with a neighbour who had also had a mastectomy several years ago. She made me feel so much better, a real sharing. Over the next few weeks she often put notes through the door. It felt as though she was with me in what I was going through.* — Vicki

- Most neighbours will appreciate being told about your ordeal so that they can offer support. Neighbours can help look after children, take you to hospital for appointments, do some shopping for you.

- Sometimes it can be easier with neighbours because you don't have to worry about protecting them as much as family and close friends. There is less emotional history and investment.

> *Barry knew our neighbours better than I did. He chats very easily with people. He told the neighbours about my cancer and I was thrilled to receive flowers and cards from them. It did not feel intrusive at all.* — Vicki

- We have already made the point that it is your choice who you tell. We can only say that we have found a great deal of comfort from a wide range of people – partners, family, friends, work colleagues and neighbours. Different people give you different things.

When I was in hospital our neighbours looked after our dog during the day so that she could remain at home. Simon found it more comforting to come home after his day at work and visiting me to the love and affection our dog gave rather than a cold and empty house. I was very touched when on my return there were some flowers and a get-well card waiting for me.

Another neighbour, whom I hadn't seen for some time, popped in to say goodbye before she moved. She asked me how I was. I hesitated before answering. She was terribly upset that we had lived next door and she hadn't known I was ill. — Jo

---

- Most neighbours will appreciate being told about your ordeal and will be willing to offer some help. They may be able to support you by looking after children, taking you to hospital for appointments, doing bits of shopping for you and so on. Even if they are unable to do anything practical to help, knowing they are concerned and wishing you well can be very uplifting.

ભૃૐૂ

When I've been recovering and on my own it has been so reassuring to know there are people in such close proximity that could help if needed. —Jo

*A Friend may well be reckoned
the masterpiece of Nature.*

Ralph Waldo Emerson (1803–82)

Choice 30

Know Your Limits

This above all: to thine own self be true.

William Shakespeare (1564–1616)
HAMLET

While you are in treatment, don't make the mistake of expecting yourself to do everything you used to do when you were well. Some treatments can drain you of energy for a time and you can easily make yourself feel even worse by forcing yourself to do more than you need.

🍃 Learn to listen and respond to your body's needs. If you feel tired, allow yourself to rest as much as possible. If you are not used to doing this you might consider including some meditation in your daily timetable. Many of us are not very aware of the things our bodies are trying to tell us. We are so busy living our lives that we have little time to stop and take stock of how we actually are. Meditation will help you become more aware of the signals your body is giving you and it will also help you to slow down and calm yourself when you are feeling anxious.

<svg>≫</svg> There are lots of different ways of meditating and no particular one is really any better than the rest. You can experiment with different techniques until you find one that suits you. Here is one way to start:

Find a place in which you can be comfortable and uninterrupted. There is no need to adopt a special position unless you want to follow a particular school of meditation. Sit in a chair which gives you good support, or on the floor if you are more comfortable there. Breathe slowly and deeply, relax the muscles of your face and jaw, and close your eyes. When you are breathing rhythmically, count as you breathe in, pause and then allow the same count for the out-breath. Let your breathing be gentle and quiet.

I wanted Vicki to go back to work as this is what she wanted but she had a responsible job and I was worried that it would be terribly hard for her. I knew it would be of benefit to her if it went well but I had fears about her being able to cope and I did not want her to get over-tired. — Barry

🐦 If you are working during this period discuss the situation with your manager and try to make an arrangement that allows you to reduce your working hours or the amount of stress, if at all possible.

I got tremendous support at work. I used to get waves of tiredness suddenly coming over me. The people I worked with seemed to know when this was happening and sent me to my mum's to have a sleep. (I worked near my parents' house.) I used to sleep for a couple of hours and go back to work. —Jo

---

🐦 Overdoing it can set you back, physically and mentally. Set targets – simple ones – and grade them according to how you feel. Check with a nurse or general practitioner to find out if these are reasonable. You can't measure tiredness but you can translate targets into concrete terms. You can always upgrade or downgrade them. Above all, listen to your body. Tiredness can be attributed to treatment but also to the aftermath of trauma.

🐦 Be reasonable with yourself. Don't push yourself too hard. You may not have the reserves of energy you had before. Feeling tired does not mean your treatment is not working. This is all part of your journey and like any journey this one has some territory that can be difficult to travel through.

Choice 31

When In Doubt, Cry!

If you have tears, prepare to shed them now.

William Shakespeare (1564–1616)
JULIUS CAESAR

Since that day I have learned to face myself. I have had to come to terms with having cancer and losing a breast and it has not been easy. For some weeks I was very vulnerable and just needed to cry to wash the pain out of my system and begin again. —Vicki

---

I found myself crying at odd times, especially when I was driving on my own. —Jo

---

There are bound to be times when your feelings are very close to the surface and you really need to let yourself go. The problem for some of us though is that we might have been brought up to believe that giving vent to feelings is bad form or a sign that we are not being brave enough. Little children, however, seem to be much wiser than we are. If you watch young children you will notice how immediately they express how they are feeling. If they are angry they shout, if they are sad they cry. Usually after a few minutes it's all over and they go on to the next bit of life.

- If you are in pain, physically or emotionally, you have every right to have a good cry. It is a natural reaction and, surprisingly, most people do feel better afterwards.

- For some people the fear that if they start weeping they will never stop prevents them from letting themselves get the feelings out of their system. You may well find that you can't stop for ages, especially if you have held everything in for a long time. Don't worry – just let yourself cry. You will stop eventually, and you will feel better for it.

- You may prefer to have a close friend with you some of the time while you cry or you may want to be on your own. If you are with someone, you can reassure that person there is no need to do anything – just having the friend there can be a great comfort.

- Remember that letting yourself go in this way is not childish or weak. No-one should feel ashamed about acknowledging and expressing true feelings.

When In Doubt, Cry!

❦

Happiness is beneficial for the body, but it is grief that develops the powers of the mind.

Marcel Proust (1871–1922)

Choice 32

Or Laugh!

The most wasted of all days is that on which one has not laughed.

Nicholas Chamford (1741–1794)

Laughing, too, is a great way to dissipate tension and fear. It might seem almost sacrilegious to laugh when you are really ill or down, but laughter can be as therapeutic as tears. In fact there is a therapy movement developing which is based on encouraging people to laugh as a way of improving their healing.

❧ You can find humour in the most unlikely places.

When I arrived at the specialist hospital I felt anxious and scared. I was feeling low when Simon left on the evening before the operation. I went to the toilet and a fellow patient asked me in the unforgettable line, 'Are you a tit or a tum?' It took time for it to click that I was in a joint gynaecological and breast cancer ward. It made me laugh and I found the humour in the ward was incredible. —Jo

Or Laugh!

❧ Make a point of switching into comedy radio or television programmes that make you laugh; go to see films which will lighten your mood; read funny books and so on. None of these will make you feel good all the time but you will get some relief even if it's only for a little while.

> *I felt having a sense of humour was really important, notwithstanding the seriousness of the situation. It's always been our policy to keep laughing, even though sometimes this was more of a reaction laugh, just like when you were in trouble at school.* — Simon

> *The anaesthetist told me her name. I said, 'My consultant has the same name as you!' 'That's because he's my husband!' she said.* —Vicki

Laughter can be helpful and therapeutic because it can give you a sense of survival rather than despair.

Jesting often cuts hard knots more effectively than gravity.

Cicero (106–43 BC)

Choice 33

Keep A Journal

I'll call for pen and ink, and write my mind.

William Shakespeare (1564–1616)
HENRY VI

Putting your thoughts and emotions on paper is a good way of getting things out and setting them in order. Keeping a journal also provides you with a record of this particular time in your life that you may want to look back on.

It doesn't matter if you've never written anything before. No-one is going to read it, unless you choose to show it to people. No-one is going to check up on your grammar or handwriting!

In creating, the only hard thing's to begin;
A grass-blade's no easier to make than an oak.
If you've once found the way, you've achieved the grand
stroke.

J.R. Lowell (1818–1891)

❧ Don't set yourself any rules like having to write every day. Just write when you feel like it.

❧ Take some care in choosing the book or paper you are going to use; decorate the cover if you wish. Make this a special book for you. If a book seems too daunting just write your notes, thoughts, feelings, one-off lines, quotations you want to keep, etc. on scraps of paper. You can collect them into a special box or file.

❧ Writing is a good way of uncluttering the confusion you may be feeling inside.

❧ You can draw pictures or symbols to describe how you feel or just jot down words or phrases. Paste in pictures that you come across which mean something to you.

❧ You might come across a particularly inspiring poem or piece of prose to include.

❧ If you would like to start but can't think how, pick up your pen (or put your hands on the keyboard) and write down whatever words come into your mind. There are only these rules: don't take your pen off the paper or your hands off the keyboard and don't make any sense. Just doodle with the words. Write steadily and enjoy it.

❧ Anything can go into your journal. You don't have to limit your thoughts or creativity. Think of your journal as your confidante and friend, someone to whom you can tell your innermost thoughts and feelings. This is a place where you can be absolutely honest with yourself.

Writing a journal had the same effect as crying – I was able to get out what I was feeling in a way that I couldn't do with anyone I know. It was also very useful to look back. I felt compelled to write, at first only for myself, then later to share with others. — Vicki

---

Although I've never kept a diary I felt a strong desire to write down my thoughts. It helped me straighten out in my mind how I was feeling. At first, when I was writing everything seemed to be a jumble but by writing it down my thoughts seemed to make more sense. — Jo

Choice 34

A Little Of What You Fancy

How you might make your life as easy and pleasant as possible during this difficult time is a theme to which we keep returning because we feel it is so important to your recovery. We want you to pamper yourself as much as possible. Here are some of the things that helped us but you will probably make your own list.

- Sit in the garden watching someone else doing the weeding!

- Start a hobby that you've always wanted to have a go at. Let it be something you can pick up and put down as you feel like it.

- Do nothing for a while.

- Meet friends.

- Go out for a meal.

- Phone for a take-away if you don't feel like cooking.

❧ Have a clothes-swap with a friend.

❧ Browse for ages in a good bookshop.

❧ Get in touch with people you haven't been in contact with for a while.

❧ Read 'happy ending' books.

❧ Listen to music you like.

❧ Light a scented candle.

❧ Ask someone to take you for a drive.

❧ Spend time looking after your body; use scented lotions, bath bubbles and so on.

❧ Take a trip down memory lane playing old records or looking at old photos.

❧ Invite friends over.

❧ Watch videos, films, television programmes that you enjoy even if they're not high culture!

Obviously how you pamper yourself depends on your own

tastes, time available and your purse. The above are the things we did to help us — you can make your own programme for pampering yourself. Try to find one thing you can do each day that you know will make you feel good, even if only briefly. Make it as important as taking your prescribed medicines.

You may feel that this is being much too selfish but in our view how you look after yourself does affect your recovery.

To love oneself is the beginning of a life-long romance.

Oscar Wilde (1856–1900)
AN IDEAL HUSBAND

Choice 35

Believe What You Believe

We have encouraged you to find help from the people around you who can be a great source of comfort and consolation. You have, however, another resource available to you and that is what is inside you!

There are certain questions that most of us ask ourselves from time to time. 'What is the meaning of life?' 'Why is this happening to me?' 'Why am I here?' 'Why is everyone else here?' We search for a meaning for what is happening to us. We try to interpret events to help us find a meaning. We use images, myths and metaphors to help us understand the meaning of life as a whole and give meaning to our experience.

Some of us are able to depend on religious beliefs, others on philosophical ideas. Many people have no such systematic belief framework but create their own way of making life meaningful. Each of us needs some way of making order in a seemingly chaotic world.

To everything there is a season, and a time to every purpose under heaven; a time to be born, and a time to die; a time to plant, and a time to pluck up that which is planted; a time to kill and a time to heal; … A time to weep, and a time to laugh; … A time to keep silence and a time to speak; a time to love and a time to hate; a time of war and a time of peace.

Ecclesiastes

This is a time to re-affirm religious or philosophical beliefs in which you have faith because they can offer comfort and support when you feel most frightened and alone. We don't have a view that any particular belief is the best or the only one. People who have a strong religious belief very often gain great solace from the practice of that religion. The notion that there is some power outside yourself can be a source of strength and inspiration.

For those who have no such beliefs, inspiration can often be obtained from the words of philosophers, artists, community leaders and so on. They can help you keep a sense of the purpose of life at times when you might be feeling most hopeless.

❧ Look for anything on which you can lean for support, grow from and enjoy: poetry, literature, inspirational writings and so on. If you are keeping a journal, they can become an important part of it.

❧ Listen to people who speak in such a way that you feel inspired by them.

Although I don't openly practise a religion I've always believed in God and this in some way helped me through. I never questioned why I had cancer; I never asked, 'Why me?' I actually thought, 'Why not me?' — Jo

---

To begin with I often thought I would find out the point of all this at some later date in a flash of revelation. But now I believe that there is no rhyme or reason. I think that this is life, everybody has ups and downs, triumphs and disasters. You just have to deal with the downs as quickly and thoroughly as possible to make way for whatever is going to happen next.

—Vicki

Faith consists in believing when it is beyond the power of reason to believe. It is not enough that a thing be possible for it to be believed.

Voltaire (1694–1778)

I am not a believer in religion but I needed something to hold on to. I looked through books to find someone who would speak to me. I got great comfort from Kahlil Gibran's 'The Prophet'.

—Vicki

Section 4 The Aftermath

'What Happens Now?'

Choice 36

On Your Own?

The time will come when your treatment has finished. You may still be on medication but you are probably now beginning to feel that you are getting your normal life back. This may come as a relief because you may have felt that for some time your life was taken over by your illness, medical appointments and treatment schedules.

Returning to your old life can also feel frightening. During your illness the world revolved around you as people concentrated on your survival and you have been the centre of attention. Now you may feel vulnerable and be wondering whether you are strong enough to manage on your own.

Let me assert my firm belief that the only thing we have to fear is fear itself.

Franklin D. Roosevelt (1882–1945)

❧ Remember that you are not entirely on your own. You can still contact the medical professionals for advice and check-ups.

﹏ You can still be in contact with those groups and organisations who have helped you with advice and information.

You can be proud of yourself for having got to this point. You have come through a very difficult stage of your illness and are ready for the next step in the journey.

Now that your treatment is finished your worst fears may be that the cancer will come back. It may help you to discuss these fears with your consultant. The days when people did not feel able to discuss cancer openly have long gone but people do vary in their wish to know details. Your consultant should be sensitive to your wishes and discuss things with you to whatever extent you want. He or she will not be able to tell you that the cancer will never return because cancer is unpredictable and it is not possible to have any guarantees.

Everyone worries about illness but living with the fear that the cancer may return means that every little ache and pain feels threatening. Even a cold can be worrying at first and you might not be able to stop yourself wondering, 'Is there something different about this cold from the colds I used to get pre-cancer?'

Whenever I have an ache or pain I wonder if a stray cell has broken free and I am afraid. I do not like uncertainty and the question 'Has it really gone?' can only be answered in a few years' time. —Vicki

I still cannot prevent myself feeling nervous every time Mum goes for her breast cancer check-ups and am always very relieved when I hear her voice on the phone saying that everything is fine. —Jillian

Some pain and symptoms such as unexpected bleeding are especially worrying but you should not hesitate to go to your GP about anything that is troubling you, however trivial it might appear. Although this is easy to say it can be incredibly difficult to pick up the phone and make an appointment and then verbalise the symptom to your doctor. It means facing it and the possible implications. You may have to contain your fears and steel yourself to function normally even though you are churning up inside thinking, 'I don't know if I can go through all this again!'

🐦 There is a limit to how much you should expect yourself to contain. The sooner you report what is happening the calmer you will feel and the sooner it can be checked.

Partners and those others who care deeply about you will also feel vulnerable when you are not well. You are something of a barometer for them – when you are well they will be content; when you are ill they will worry about you.

> *I'm continually observing Vicki. I am much more aware of illness and the worst scenarios.* — Barry

> *I'm glad Jo is under constant monitoring – I feel that she is being carefully looked after.* — Cyril

> *I find that when I ask Jo 'How are you?' it is no longer one of those cliché questions you ask people. I listen very carefully for the answer, trying to gauge from her tone or the particular words she uses whether everything really is OK.* — Sheila

Fear usually becomes easier to manage as time goes on but the anxiety can hang around for a long time and may never entirely go. You may even find yourself worrying about not feeling anxious. It can be hard to feel safe and confident after all that you have been through.

What is worth remembering is that it is natural to feel anxious about the cancer returning. Even if you had not had cancer you might worry if you became ill or developed an unusual symptom. What is different now is that there is a shadow with which you have to live. If you feel overwhelmed with anxiety from time to time, look again at Choice 19.

> *As time moves on I don't feel the panic anymore when I go for routine monitoring tests but anything out of the ordinary still worries me.* — Jo

Choice 37

The World Of Check-ups

Although your treatment has finished and you are able to resume your normal life you will doubtless be returning to hospital for regular check-ups. The irony is that the first few check-ups are the most anxiety provoking but you need them for peace of mind and the security they offer. After that, as time goes on, you will feel more confident and the check-ups become part of your progress towards a normal life.

Your consultant will decide how often you need to be seen. It might be monthly at first, then three monthly, six monthly and then an annual check-up.

Monitoring is often a long-term programme and can last for 10 years. It is there for your benefit. Your consultant can find out how you are getting on and you can ask any questions you may have about your condition.

However, these check-ups bring up a mixture of emotions. Each one reminds you of the ordeal you have undergone. You may be really frightened with questions like, 'What are they going to find this time? What will they tell me?' going round in your mind. The process of having to go for regular checks can be a drain, especially if all you want to do is get on with your life.

Your check-up may consist of a variety of procedures. There is likely to be a physical examination and there may also be X-rays, scans, ultra-sound and blood tests.

> *I slept badly as I was terrified about my bone scan, liver ultra sound, chest X-ray and mammogram taking place the next day. It was a year after my mastectomy and I was waiting in limbo all over again. I worried myself sick about what the consultant was going to tell me. I was quite overcome when he told me three days later that I was fine. It was just wonderful.* —Vicki

Those close to you will also be anxious about your check-ups.

> *It's always an anxious time when Vicki has her scans and check-ups although the consultant is very reassuring each time. I've always felt confident although at the back of my mind are the questions 'Will there be something wrong? Will the cancer have spread?'* —Barry

> *There is always going to be a lurking fear that a result is going to come out and not be what is wanted, so part of me steels myself for the worst.* — Alisa

Gradually your check-ups will feel easier as your confidence in your body returns, although some anxiety will probably always be there. Treat yourself each time you complete a check-up. You deserve it!

Your worst fears can be realised if the cancer returns. It may be a local recurrence reappearing in the same part of your body or it may appear somewhere else. Because cancer is so unpredictable, your doctors may not know why the cancer has returned. Cancer not caught at an early stage is more likely to return; some types of cancer are more likely to spread than others.

- The recurrence may be as bad or even worse than the original and you may be tempted to lose faith in your own ability to fight or lose confidence in the people treating you.

But you must remember that:

- A recurrence does not mean that you will not overcome it; some people have several recurrences and go on to recover completely. Don't let your disappointment make you give up.

> *I found it encouraging to see that other people who had been diagnosed with cancer were still around and getting on with their lives.* —Jo

🖎 Treat yourself kindly. It might take longer this time to adjust to all that is involved in treating your cancer. Most of the medical procedures will be familiar to you although your treatment might be different this time. You may find it exhausting but you will cope and go on to fight your cancer again.

If you know the enemy and know yourself, you need not fear the result of a hundred battles.

Sun Tzu

Choice 38

Stepping Into Your Future

Once your treatment has finished you will be thinking about taking up your normal life. The balance of your life changed when you knew you had cancer. It was the cancer and all it meant that weighed the scales down but now the balance is changing again. The scales are coming down on the side of normality again.

Although you are ready to resume your old life, things might never feel quite the same again. You have faced a frightening and painful predicament and this experience may have changed how you look at life quite profoundly.

❧ In some ways time will have stood still for other people while you have been fighting to survive. Some will be very anxious to know how you are feeling, others will want to regard you as cured and some may want to avoid you because they do not know what to say. People are likely to want to take their cue from you so if you are open about your illness they will be open too; if you don't want to talk about it they will probably avoid the topic. On the other hand, you might meet someone whom you haven't seen for some time and who may not know you have had cancer.

> *The way Jo was so honest and open about her feelings gave me the strength and courage to face my own.* — Alisa

❧ Getting back to normal might mean that you now have to make some important decisions which had been put on hold throughout your illness. These will have a new impetus if you are worried about continuing to be well enough to carry them out. Another possibility is that your illness has brought about changes with regard to what you want in your life and you may wish to rethink decisions in the light of this. Take time so that you can be certain you are considering all the options and making decisions you will be satisfied to live with.

> *My decision to carry on with the fertility treatment was mind-blowing. I guess I'll never know if it was the right decision but it was the only one I could live with.* — Jo

> *Even pre-cancer, however unhappy I was with my work, Jo encouraged me to make changes. I found it hard to follow my dreams but, post-cancer, Jo has shown me how fragile life can*

be. It has enabled me to take a gamble and start up on my own in business. —Simon

- If you have had a long absence from work you may be keen to return but apprehensive about how you will be able to pick up your job again, as well as feeling vulnerable about your health. Try not to expect yourself to take up exactly where you left off. As we have already said you are not really in the same place as you were before the cancer. Don't be disappointed if you can't fit in straight away; take time to settle yourself back into your working life.

- What has happened to you may be affecting some of your colleagues for whom your illness has made them face up to their own mortality. They could also be worrying that if job stress was implicated in your cancer, they, too, may succumb to the disease. We all deal with our anxieties in different ways, so you may be bewildered by the reactions you might notice from the people around you. Some colleagues may want to talk about your illness, perhaps more that you would like; others will apparently ignore it altogether, treating you as if nothing had happened. Probably it's true to say that the more open you are about your feelings and thoughts, the easier others will find it to communicate. But don't put yourself under the pressure of talking about things you would rather keep to yourself.

I never expected Jo to suffer illness; she and I were used to being strong. In fact we did not tolerate illness in any way! Now my attitude has completely changed because of Jo's experience. I am now far more tolerant and caring toward people I work with. I still wonder how long Jo's body was developing the cancer and hope that I did not contribute to it! — Anne

Although you may want to put the cancer behind you, fears may intrude into your working life and you may even have occasional flashbacks.

On one occasion I was at a training day where participants were told to close their eyes and imagine Health and Social Services in 20 years' time. I was in tears – I could not imagine being alive in 20 years. The fear of cancer was all around me and this was particularly distressing in a work environment although people were very understanding. — Vicki

Returning to work is an important part of your recovery and a good support network will help smooth your passage. It may or may not be possible and appropriate for you to share some of your feelings of vulnerability with your colleagues. How you make the choice will depend on the culture in your particular organisation. Our experience is that colleagues appreciated openness because it demonstrated how possible it was to have cancer and come through it. We also felt helped and supported by their willingness to discuss these things. If you do not want to talk about your cancer at work you may feel like finding another outlet so that you can express your thoughts and feelings to someone rather than keeping them inside yourself.

Choice 39

You Can Be Strong

Living with the aftermath of cancer can be hard. There are times when, however well you are dealing with things, you somehow get ambushed by situations you can't predict. For instance, you might hear of someone you know having a recurrence of cancer or read in the paper of a well-known person dying after struggling with cancer. It's hard not to respond to the news by thinking, 'That could be me,' and experiencing again those fearful feelings with which you have became familiar …

But you are not the same person that you were before you had cancer. Your experience has changed and strengthened you. You have faced and may still be facing one of the greatest fears human beings can have. Give yourself credit for coming this far.

One of the days I was feeling particularly down at work, a colleague told me out of the blue that I was an inspiration to him by the fact that I'd actually continued working. This really perked me up. —Jo

Cancer changes you inside even if you look just the same on the outside. We think it is worth considering how you can use the strength you have developed as a result.

> *Of all existing things some are in our power and others are not in our power. In our power are thought, impulse, will to get and will to avoid, and in a word, everything which is our own doing.*

Epictetus (60–120)

Here are some suggestions:

- You might want to use your experience to help others who are going through the same ordeal. One way of doing this is to become a volunteer for one of the cancer organisations, either helping with administration or talking to people who want to speak with someone who has had a similar experience to them. Some organisations offer special training. They might want to check out with you that you have adjusted to having cancer yourself so that your own experience will not get in the way of helping others.

- You can talk to people informally. You may find that family and acquaintances will ask you to have a chat with someone they know who has been diagnosed with cancer.

I had known Jo for many years as our families had lived near each other and were friends. I was shocked when she was diagnosed with ovarian cancer. She was so young and had her life in front of her. I was able to help Jo by listening to her and giving her some leaflets to read. We developed a close relationship that I have really valued. — Vicki

❧ You may not feel like talking to people but there are other ways of helping. Many cancer sufferers raise money for cancer causes. They want to give something back to those who have helped them and hopefully make things better for people who in the future will be diagnosed with cancer. Thousands of pounds have been raised in this way by ordinary people and celebrities.

❧ Most cancer organisations welcome volunteers and you can become involved in a wide range of activities, depending on what interests you. You might, for instance, be interested in the public relations side.

I was interviewed for two magazines on the way people are told that they have cancer and other aspects of cancer from the lay person's point of view. Then Bacup had a press conference and asked me to speak as a user of their services. This was daunting but exciting too. — Vicki

❧ Finally you might even think of setting up a cancer support group.

> *I worked for a local authority and was aware of other women in the organisation with breast cancer. I set up a breast cancer support group. It was the first workplace cancer support group in the country and ran for two years.* — Vicki

Choice 40

Stop Looking For Blame

Cancers develop because something affects the normal way that cells in a particular part of the body divide and reproduce. There are many theories as to why this happens. Some people think that the environment is to blame; others that diet is the cause. There are theories that cancer sometimes follows a life crisis such as bereavement or divorce; stress has also been implicated as a factor. However, researchers still need to find out more about the processes that occur in the cells during the development of different types of cancer to be really sure as to the cause.

It is natural for us to try to find reasons for things that happen to us. Maybe we feel that the more we can understand the more we can feel in control. People with cancer often feel that they have caused the illness themselves and may torture themselves with the thought that if they had done something differently they would not be in this situation.

I returned and saw under the sun, that the race is not to the swift, nor the battle to the strong, neither yet bread to the wise, nor yet riches to men of understanding, nor yet favour to men of skill; but time and chance happeneth to them all.

Ecclesiastes 9:11–12

❧ Feeling guilty or looking for who is to blame will not solve or change anything. If you doubt this try setting a timer for five minutes. Then for the next five minutes make yourself feel as guilty as you possible can. When the timer rings for the end of the five minutes ask yourself, 'What has changed?' Nothing will have changed, except that you might be feeling even worse.

❧ Something with which the experts seem to agree is that many factors are involved in getting cancer. One way of thinking about it is to imagine that we are like those machine games in which a combination of different elements have to come up before it will pay out the money. There's no point in blaming the machine or the player for not bringing up the winning combinations – it's a matter of chance. In our bodies, a particular combination of factors may come up with the 'payoff' of cancer and, similarly, there's no point in blaming yourself for this. You did not set out to get cancer — it happened because a number of factors of which you are unaware, or which are outside your control, came together.

If you find yourself troubled by guilty thoughts about the past or worries about what might happen in the future, concentrate instead on the present and how you might make the best of what you have.

I know without a shadow of doubt that the cancer has had an extremely positive effect. I am much more laid back about life. I try so hard not to get stressed; easier said than done, of course. I try not to put off things that I want to do, until tomorrow, or delay things that I don't want to do until next month! — Jo

Choice 41

Genes: To Test Or Not

In most cases cancer is not inherited or passed down through families. However, in a small number of families it is thought that a faulty gene might make some people more likely to get breast, bowel or ovarian cancer.

A gene change is suspected when a number of women in the same family have developed breast or ovarian cancer, particularly if this has occurred at a young age. However, if you have a genetic fault it is not certain that you will develop cancer. It just increases the likelihood. It is possible to have a test to find out if you are carrying a faulty gene that could result in breast or ovarian cancer. The test is only suggested if there is a family history of these types of cancer. It is not conclusive as only certain genes have been identified and you may have an alteration in a gene as yet unknown so it cannot always guarantee peace of mind.

If you have this test and it turns out to be positive, you have some difficult decisions to make. Research suggests that having both breasts removed may reduce the risk of breast cancer and having a hysterectomy and ovaries removed will avoid the risk of ovarian cancer. However, these are drastic steps to take and other alternatives such as regular screening and drug treatment can be discussed with medical professionals.

- Before embarking on a genes test you do need to consider all the implications. Most hospitals will not do this test until some counselling has taken place.

- For some people living with uncertainty is more painful than knowing as much as possible about their situation. However, of course, this is a choice that only you can make for yourself.

I decided to have a genes test as there is a lot of breast cancer in my family. I discussed the implications with my daughters because if I had a faulty gene then they might have inherited it too. They wanted me to go ahead. My test was clear but it is still possible that I may have an alteration in another gene yet to be identified. I felt very emotional having the genes test done and it was difficult waiting for the results but I wanted my daughters and grand-daughters to feel as safe as possible.

— Vicki

Mum's breast cancer, along with several close relatives also having breast cancer on her side of the family, highlighted a likely genetic link. This means that I will be screened every

> *year for breast cancer from the age of 35. Screening makes me*
> *feel anxious but I think it is something positive I can do to*
> *make sure that I stay healthy.* —Laura

Apart from genes tests there are other tests which can be done to find out if you are likely to develop cancers. There are some other cancers which can be tested for in this way. For example a test can be carried out to detect the likelihood of bowel cancer which is offered to families where there has been a history of bowel cancer.

- Be aware that you often have to declare gene testing on insurance applications.

Remember …

You know yourself better than anyone else, so in the end only you can know whether you will be more anxious knowing or not knowing the likely risk of developing cancer. Whether or not to take a test is your choice and whatever you choose to do will be right for you.

> *I chose not to be tested because of the implications it would*
> *have for my family, although if I do have children I'm sure I*
> *will then have the test.* —Jo

Choice 42

Time To Take Stock

Having cancer can bring about many changes. This may be the point in your cancer journey for you to evaluate what has happened to you.

> You may find your view of life changed as a result of your experiences.

Personally I'm much more relaxed at work now. This doesn't mean I don't get stressed but I don't fret about not meeting impossible deadlines any more. —Jo

---

I have survived one of my worst fears. It has given me the courage to feel that I can face anything. —Vicki

---

I feel both of us now show a lot more courage. We do not just talk about plans; we get on and do them. I now understand how fragile the gift of life is and how easily it can be taken away. —Simon

❧ Your priorities may have changed.

> *For many years I felt I was wasting my life, being stuck in a rut and not taking any care of myself, but over the last couple of years I'm beginning to achieve what I always wanted to. Ironically, if Jo had never got cancer there's a high chance I'd still be in that rut.* — Simon

> *We have good holidays and don't worry about saving money for our old age too much. We have worked hard and want to spend money on ourselves. Thinking back, it was a very traumatic time but we coped with it very well. We make better use of our lives now, knowing things can go wrong.* — Barry

❧ Relationships can take on a new meaning.

> *Jo's experience has made me appreciate my good health and not take anything about the future for granted. Although we were good friends before, if anything Jo's experience has brought us closer together.* — Laura

> *Vicki's operation was a great success and there's been no detrimental effect on our life together. It has not affected our sexual relationship and has made us much closer and appreciative of each other. We know we can trust each other to be supportive.* — Barry

I look at Jo in a new light. I always thought highly of how she copes with difficult situations. This, though, has really impressed me, if that is the right word. I suspect she found she was capable of more than she thought she could expect of herself. — Cyril

I was pregnant at the time I came over to visit Jo. She never once gave me an uncomfortable feeling and always asked me lots of questions about the baby, not because she had to but really because she was interested and worried about me. I thought she was amazing! And no words at the moment could describe how much I love her. — Alisa

The best thing to have come out of this experience has been the strengthening of our partnership not just in love but in friendship and the knowledge that we are now always there for each other, whatever may come. — Simon

Life is mostly froth a bubble;
Two things stand like stone,
Kindness in another's trouble,
Courage in your own.

Adam Lindsay Gordon (1833–70)

Choice 43

❦

Do You Want To Make Changes?

Unceasingly contemplate the generation of all things through change, and accustom thyself to the thought that the Nature of the Universe delights above all in changing the things that exist and making new ones of the same pattern. For everything that exists is the seed of that which shall come out of it.

Marcus Aurelius (121–180)

Having taken stock of what has happened, you might well decide to make some changes in your life. Having cancer can help you see what is important and what is not. You may make new goals for your life.

- ❧ You may want to treat your body more carefully, take more exercise, treat yourself to a massage, eat more healthily and so on.

- ❧ You may try to let go of some bad feelings from the past.

I had no contact with my divorced husband who left me for a close friend. Although I have a happy life with a loving partner I had never been able to forgive my ex-husband for making me suffer and my feelings about him had been left largely unresolved. I decided to try and overcome my resentment and met my ex-husband for lunch. We talked for several hours and in doing so I managed to confront my feelings and let go of some of the past. — Vicki

> You may want to write about your cancer experience. This can help you to let go of what you are feeling and also help other people by telling them about your experience and what has helped you.

One thing that has been amazing is the process of writing this book. To actually hear how my partner, family and friends were feeling about my having cancer has been incredible. I guess without asking directly I would never have known how deeply everyone around me has been affected. — Jo

Writing about my cancer has been important to me. It has enabled me to share my experience in a different way with those closest to me. — Vicki

❧ The most important thing is that you make the choice yourself. Some people are able to see their cancer as a positive influence in helping them sort out their lives.

I am no longer afraid to look forward, to take risks, to enjoy myself. I now believe I will be alive for a good few years but if in the unlikely event that I am not I am making sure that I don't waste this life and feel regret for things never done. Until I had cancer that is exactly how I felt. — Jo

---

❧ Keep devising goals: big ones, small ones, short-term and long-term. Don't be afraid to drop one if it doesn't suit you, or if you change your mind, or if it turns into a Pyrrhic victory. It won't be the 'be all and end all'. Stay objective. Not achieving your goals doesn't mean you've failed or that you couldn't do it because of the cancer.

❧ Make a list of things you would like to do. Include everything you can think of, however fantastic it may seem. This can be the first step towards creating the kind of life you want. When you have made your list, put it away for a period of time and then look at it. You may be pleasantly surprised at how much you can achieve.

❧

When I was first diagnosed I made a list of what I would like to achieve.

1. *Become a mother*
2. *Actively work for a charity*
3. *Make more time for social activities*
4. *Write a book*
5. *Work part-time*
6. *Get in touch with old friends*
7. *Lose weight*
8. *Read more*

I only rediscovered this list recently and was amazed that much of it has been completed. — Jo

❧ It is also true that although your life priorities may change, this might only be a temporary change and you may decide that you want life to go on just as it was before. The choice is yours. Whatever you decide to do will be right for you.

There is a certain relief in change, even though it be from bad to worse; as I have found in travelling in a stage-coach, it is often a comfort to shift one's position and be bruised in a new place.

Washington Irving (1783–1859)

Choice 44

Celebrate Your Living

Today, whatever may annoy,
The word for me is Joy, just simple Joy.

John Kendrick Bangs (1862–1922)

You have journeyed this far through your experience of cancer and are now ready to face the next part of your life. It isn't possible to know with certainty what lies ahead but we feel that this moment is worth celebrating.

- Some celebrations are inward. You may find that you value everyday life more. A beautiful summer day, for instance, can take on a new meaning. A day spent in the garden; reading an enjoyable book; going to the hairdresser; doing the shopping; a day in the office; meeting friends – all these very ordinary activities can be celebrations of your good feeling about yourself.

- You may decide to write a poem, take a trip abroad – anything which has meaning for you and will be a marker for your achievement.

❧ You may choose to celebrate by marking a particular date that has meaning for you each year.

We now have an extra anniversary to celebrate. This is November 6th, the day that Vicki was diagnosed with cancer. Each time it's another year gone by. It has given us another anniversary which is as important as birthdays. — Barry

---

❧ You may want to celebrate with the friends and family who have been on this journey with you. You might hold a party or invite some people to a special meal.

When I was diagnosed with cancer a close friend came to comfort me and through my tears told me that we would celebrate our 60th birthdays together. Six years later we had a wonderful joint celebration. — Vicki

---

❧ Be kind to those around you – and let them be kind to you.

Choice 44½

Our Last Word

Our aim in this book has been to show you that you do have choices where you might have felt you had none. We have tried to accompany you as you have travelled through your cancer journey. We have come to the end of the book even though you may still be in the middle of your own personal journey. This last choice is only a half one because none of us can really choose how long we are going to live. We can only choose what we do with the life we have in front of us.

Whatever choices you make:

- Be kind to yourself. Try taking up the suggestions we have made throughout the book as to how you can look after yourself during this time. You are the most important person to yourself and the only one who really knows how you are feeling and what you need. Staying in touch with yourself will help you make the most of life.

- Be kind to those around you. The people who care

about you are no doubt doing their best to help you through this time. As you will have seen from the quotations, family and friends also experience pain and anxiety. Being honest and open with them will ensure that you do not have to make this journey alone.

- Take each day as it comes. Although the past is always with us in our memories and we need to think about the future in order to make plans, in fact the present is what we actually have now. Make the most of it.

- Accept how you feel. There is no right way to feel about having cancer. However you feel is right for that moment.

One thing I have noticed is that emotionally I am still very up and down. There are times when I feel very fragile and times when I feel very confident. I realise that life will never be the same as it was before I had cancer. — Jo

---

Glossary

Anaesthetist A person trained to administer anaesthetics.

Anaesthetic – local A drug, cream or injection to make part of your body temporarily numb.

Anaesthetic – general A drug that puts you to sleep while you undergo an operation or procedure.

Benign Describes a tumour or growth that is not cancerous.

Biopsy The removal of a sample of tissue so that it can be examined in the laboratory to find the cause of an illness.

Cancer The name given to a group of diseases that can occur in any organ of the body and which involves abnormal or uncontrolled growth of cells.

Chemotherapy A cancer treatment involving a special mix of anti-cancer drugs.

CT scan Produces a cross-section image of the head and body which is then analysed by computer.

Gene Units of inheritance carrying the chemical blue-prints for correct cell reproduction.

Glossary

❧❦❧

Hysterectomy The surgical removal of the uterus which can include the cervix, fallopian tubes and ovaries.

Laparoscopy A minor operation which involves making a small incision in the abdomen so that a small microscope (laparoscope) can be inserted to enable the abdomen to be examined.

MRI (Magnetic Resonance Imaging) Scan Uses radio rather than x-rays to produce pictures which are then analysed by computer.

Malignant Describes a growth or tumour that is cancerous and can grow and spread.

Mammogram A specialist x-ray which shows up the breast tissue and can detect breast cancer at an early stage.

Mastectomy The removal by surgery of all or part of the breast.

Oncology The branch of medicine that deals with the study and treatment of cancer.

Oncologist A doctor who specialises in the treatment of cancer. A clinical oncologist or radiotherapist deals with treatment with radiation, and a medical oncologist specialises in treatment with drugs.

Prognosis An assessment of the expected future course and outcome of a person's disease.

Radiotherapy The treatment of cancer by x-rays or gamma rays to destroy cancer cells.

Registrar Middle-ranking hospital doctor.

Surgery An operation.

Tumour A growth or lump which may or may not be cancerous.

Ultrasound scan Use of sound waves to build up an image of internal organs.

X-ray High energy radiation used in high doses to treat cancer or in low doses to diagnose the disease. Abnormal growths show up darker than normal organs.

Helpful Organisations

Anti-Breast & Cervical Cancer Information Service Strathmore
VIC 3041
Tel: 03 9374 3233

Breast Cancer Book Service
PO Box 449
Heidelberg
VIC 3084
Tel: 03 9457 5977

Breast Cancer Network Australia
31 Pelham Street
Carlton
VIC 3053
Tel: 03 9805 2500

Cancer Care Centre Incorporated
76 Edmund Avenue
Unley
SA 5061
Tel: 08 8272 2411

Cancer Council NSW
153 Dowling Street
Woolloomooloo
NSW 2011
Tel: 02 9334 1900

Cancer Council of the Northern Territories
Unit 3 Casi House
23 Vanderlin Drv
Casuarina
NT 810
Tel: 08 8927 4888

Cancer Self Help Group Inc
50 Carey Street
Bardon
QLD 4065
Tel: 07 3368 1245

Canhelp Cancer Support Group Inc
262 Pitt Street
Sydney
NSW 2000
Tel: 02 9264 4106

Gynaecological Cancer Society of Queensland
100 Kilkivan Avenue

Kenmore
QLD 4069
Tel: 07 3878 4790

SOUTH AFRICA

Cancer Care Centre

The Cancer Care Centre provides reflexology, aroma-therapy and grief and bereavement counselling. Home care is also offered.

63 St Andrews Drive
Durban North 4051
Tel: 031 563 1330

CanSA

The Cancer Information Service of South Africa offers much the same services as BACUP in the UK, but also has an extensive collection of specialised books which can be loaned on a two week basis. There are many CanSA offices around the country.

National Office
PO Box 2121
Bedfordview 2008
Tel: 011 616 7662
Fax: 011 616 7785

37a Main Road Mowbray 7700
PO Box 186 Rondebosch 7700

Tel: 27 21 689 5381
Fax: 27 21 689 1840
Toll free (RSA only): 0800 226622

Coping with Cancer Creatively
A four-day programme offered by Dalene Jordaan focuses on group work with art and music therapies, counselling, massage and diet.
PO Box 20 107
Durban North 4016
Tel: 031 563 5868
Fax: 031 563 7414

The Healing Association of South Africa
10 Holstead Gardens
Durban 4001
Tel/Fax: 031 90 1434

Your Cancer Connection
Sister Gill Smith runs a seven-week cancer support programme for groups and individuals, offering information, relaxation, guided imagery, managing stress and life skills.
50 Stella Road
Plumstead 7800
Tel: 021 761 4698
e-mail: gillfarris@hotmail.com

Wellness Support Group

Five-day courses focusing on immune enhancement taught around the country by Dr Margo de Kooker and Larise du Plessis.

PO Box 752292

Gardenview 2047

Tel/Fax: 011 728 5678

UNITED KINGDOM

BACUP

Helps people with cancer, their families and friends live with cancer. Specialist cancer nurses provide information, emotional support and practical advice by telephone and letter. A range of free publications and a magazine are available. Professional counsellors provide face-to-face counselling free of charge and in confidence in London and Glasgow.

3 Bath Place

Rivington Street

London EC2A 3JR

Freephone, Cancer Information Service: 0800 18 1199 (Mon–Fri 9am–7pm

Cancer Counselling Service London: 020 7696 9000 (Mon–Fri 9am–5.30pm)

Cancer Counselling Service Glasgow: 01411 553 1553 (Mon–Fri 9am–5.30pm)

Textphone available: BACUP

website: www.cancerbacup.org.uk

Breast Cancer Care

Offers practical advice, information and support to women (and their partners, families and friends) who are concerned about breast cancer. Its services include a wide range of booklets, leaflets and audiotapes, a prosthesis fitting service and one-to-one emotional support from volunteers who have themselves experienced breast cancer.

Kiln House
210 New Kings Road
London SW6 ANZ
Nationwide freeline: 0500 245 345 (Mon–Fri 10am–7pm)

Bristol Cancer Help Centre

Offers a healing programme that deals with the whole person and is complementary to medical treatment. People affected by cancer are offered relaxation, healing, visualisation, counselling, nutrition, meditation, music and art therapy. The Centre runs one-day courses, a residential week and follow-up days. A charge is made for the services, but discretionary bursaries are available.

Grove House
Cornwallis Grove
Clifton
Bristol BS8 4PG
Helpline: 0117 980 9505

British Association for Counselling

The umbrella membership body for counselling in the UK and,

as such, the standard-setting association to which all its members adhere, providing support and protection for members of the public who may seek counselling. Provides information on counselling services available locally.

1 Regent Place
Rugby
Warwickshire CV21 2PJ
Information line: 01788 578328

Cancerlink

Provides emotional support and information in response to telephone enquiries and letters on all aspects of cancer, from people with cancer, their families, friends and professionals working with them. Supports self-help groups throughout Britain and helps people who set up new groups. Free publications and audiotapes in seven languages.

11–21 Northdown Street
London N1 9BN
Freephone Cancer Information Helpline: 0800 132905
Textphone available
Freephone Asian Cancer Information Helpline: 0800 590415

Carers National Association

Offers information and support to people caring for relatives and friends. The association has branches all over the UK which are run by carers and can refer carers to local sources of help and support.

20–25 Glasshouse Yard
London EC1A 4JS
Carers line: 0345 573369 (Mon–Fri 10am–12am and 2pm–4pm)

Institute of Complementary Medicine

The institute supplies information on qualified complementary practitioners, on complementary teaching institutions and on complementary medicine generally for use by the media. Enquirers are asked to supply an SAE and two loose stamps
PO Box 194
London SE16 1QZ
Tel: 020 7237 5165

Macmillan Cancer Relief

National charity working to improve the treatment and care of people with cancer and their families from the point of diagnosis involving specialist Macmillan nurses, Macmillan doctors, buildings for cancer treatment and care, grants for patients in financial difficulties. Information on Macmillan services is available through the national Macmillan Information Line.
Anchor House
15–19 Britten Street
London SW3 3TZ
Tel: 020 7351 7811
Macmillan Information Line: 0845 601 6161 (Mon–Fri 9.30am–4.30pm)

Helpful Organisations

❧

Marie Curie Cancer Care

Provides practical hands-on nursing care at home and specialist multi-disciplinary care through its 11 Marie Curie Centres throughout the UK. Services are free to cancer patients.

28 Belgrave Square
London SW1X 8QG

The National Cancer Alliance

National membership organisation made up of users of cancer services (patients and lay carers), health professionals and other concerned individuals or groups affected by cancer. Aims to represent the interests, concerns and views of cancer patients and campaigns to ensure that high quality national standards of treatment and care are available.

PO Box 579
Oxford OX4 1LB
Tel: 01865 793566

Ovacome

A nation-wide support group for all those concerned with ovarian cancer, involving sufferers, families, friends, carers and health professionals. It aims to share personal experiences, link sufferers using the Fone Friends telephone support network, provide information on treatments, screening and research and raise awareness of the condition.

c/o St Bartholomews Hospital
West Smithfield

London EC1A 7BE
Tel: 07071 781 861 (mobile rates)
    01803 850608

New Zealand
Cancer Society of New Zealand
Regional support networks can assist people with cancer with activities such as driving, gardening, meal preparation and with support groups.
PO Box 1724
Auckland
Tel: 09 308 0162
Freephone: 0800 800 426
website: www.cancernz.org.nz

CanTeen
Peer-based support network for teenagers with cancer or life-threatening blood disorders, and for their teenage brothers and sisters.
PO Box 56 072
Dominion Road
Auckland
Tel: 09 630 3340
Fax: 09 630 3349
Freephone: 0800 226 8336
website: www.canteen.org.nz

❧

Child Cancer Foundation
PO Box 152
Auckland
Tel: 09 373 3670
Fax: 09 373 3673
website: www.childcancer.org.nz

New Zealand Breast Cancer Foundation
Tel: 09 522 4648
Fax: 09 522 4649
Freephone: 0800 902 732
website: www.breast.co.nz

REPUBLIC OF IRELAND
ARC Cancer Support Centre
Standing for Aftercare, Research and Counselling, ARC Cancer Support Centre is a voluntary organisation and registered charity which offers support to people affected by cancer, no matter where they live or where they are having their cancer treatment. This support is holistic and complements the primary medical treatment with education and psychological care. The services offered may vary from time to time and all other services are provided free of charge.
ARC House
65 Eccles Street
Dublin 7

Drop-In Service Mon. to Thurs. 10am–4.30pm
Tel: 01 830 7333
Fax: 01 830 7595
email: arc@clubi.ie

Bray Cancer Support and Information Centre
Offers emotional and practical support to people who have or
had cancer and their families. Services include a telephone
support service, social activities, home and hospital visiting and
a drop-in centre.
36B Main Street
Bray
Co. Wicklow
Tel: 01 286 6966 (24-hour answering service)

CANTEEN
Support group for adolescents who have or have had cancer,
their friends, brothers or sisters. Organises meetings, weekends
away and publishes a newsletter.
Carmichael House
North Brunswick Street
Dublin 7
Tel: 01 872 5550

Greystones Cancer Support
Offers support to cancer patients, their families and friends.
Services include hospital visiting, transport to hospital, invalid

aids, nursing equipment and monthly information meetings.
La Touche Place
Greystones
Co. Wicklow
Tel: 01 287 1601

Irish Cancer Society
5 Northumberland Road
Dublin 4
Cancer Helpline Freefone: 1800 200 700

SLÁNÚ
Cancer Help Centre
Slánú offers a programme of healing for the whole person. The various approaches of the programme are holistic and inter-connected, complementing orthodox medical practice. A five-day residential programme offers support, education and guidance. A drop-in centre and helpline service provide crisis counselling and advice, as well as private, one-to-one counselling. The Slánú support groups meet once a month. Clients are asked to contribute according to their ability to pay.
Uggool
Moycullen
Co. Galway
Tel: 091 555898
Fax: 091 555894

Turning Point

Turning Point provides a range of services, offering an integrated approach to healing, for people with a serious illness or any major life crisis. It was the first centre in Ireland to pioneer a holistic approach to the psychological care of cancer patients. All the therapies and activities at the centre are complementary to treatments prescribed by General Practitioners and Medical Specialists/Consultants.

23 Crofton Road
Dun Laoghaire
Co. Dublin
Tel: 01 280 7888/280 0626
Fax: 01 280 0643

Recommended Reading List

Dawson, Donna, *Women's Cancers*, London: Piatkus 1990
Explains cervical, breast, ovarian and endometrial cancer.

Kent, Ann, *Life After Cancer*, London: Ward Lock 1996
Practical self-help book for people whose cancer treatment has finished.

Kfir, Nira and Slevin, Maurice, *Challenging Cancer: From Chaos to Control*, London: Tavistock/Routledge 1991
For people who have been diagnosed with cancer, their families and friends. Examines feelings and emotions with the help of a psychotherapist and a cancer doctor. Suggests ways people can regain control of their lives.

Siegel, Bernie, *Living, Loving and Healing*, London: HarperCollins 1993
A book about living positively with a life-threatening disease, drawing on a wide range of spiritual, religious and psychological themes.

Simonton, Carl O., *et al*, *Getting Well Again*, London: Bantam 1986
Self-help techniques for learning positive attitudes, relaxation, visualisation.

Speechley, Val and Rosenfield, Maxine, *Cancer Information At Your Fingertips; the comprehensive cancer reference book for the 1990s*, 2nd edn, London: Class 1996
Questions and answers about cancer.

BACUP produces booklets on 'Understanding Cancer', 'Understanding Treatment' and 'Living with Cancer'.

Cancerlink produces booklets, which focus on the psychological and emotional aspects of coping with cancer.